PSYCHWARD

PSYCHWARD

A YEAR BEHIND LOCKED DOORS

STEPHEN B. SEAGER, M.D.

G. P. PUTNAM'S SONS
NEW YORK

G. P. Putnam's Sons
Publishers Since 1838
200 Madison Avenue
New York, NY 10016

Library of Congress Cataloging-in-Publication Data
Seager, Stephen B.
Psychward : a year behind locked doors / Stephen B. Seager.
p.   cm.
ISBN 0–399–13608–8
1. Seager, Stephen B.   2. Interns (Medicine)—California—Los
Angeles County—Biography.   3. Psychiatry—Study and teaching
(Internship)—California—Los Angeles County.   I. Title.
RC438.6.S43A3   1991   90–49911 CIP
616.89'0071'179493—dc20

Printed in the United States of America

1   2   3   4   5   6   7   8   9   10

This book is printed on acid-free paper.

∞

As always, to my loving wife and
three wonderful children.
To Andy and Nancy.
To my parents.
To Florence Feiler and Lisa Wager.
But especially for my late father-in-law,
Wayne. Keep on riding.

CONTENTS

Inasmuch as you have done it to the least of these my friends, you have done it unto me.

Jesus Christ
—Matt. 25:40

FOREWORD

I SUPPOSE I should say I've been a practicing psychiatrist for years. But I haven't. Or that I've been a firsthand eyewitness to the radical evolution of psychiatry over the last two decades. But that wouldn't be true, either. I am a physician, as are all psychiatrists, but I came to the profession from a different route than most. For nine years I was an emergency room doctor, a critical care specialist. The teeming ER of a big city trauma center was my home. Gunshot wounds, stabbings, overdoses, and heart attacks were my daily stock in trade. I have agonized all too frequently as people died directly beneath my hands. And felt the exultation of fanning a small, remaining flicker of life back into a flame. I have cradled beating human hearts in my fingers and picked fresh blood from the corners of my eyeglasses. I could handle the razor-sharp, face-to-face death battles with the best of them. I thought I understood what real medicine was all about, what people were all about, what being a doctor was all about. I thought I understood myself. I thought I understood a lot of things back then. Back before everything came crashing down.

I speak as if I am a psychiatrist but I am not, at least not yet. I am nearing the end of my formal training, my residency, at a sprawling, drafty mental hospital in Los Angeles, California. Officially it is known as "County General." On the street it's simply called "The Bin."

The hospital serves those who populate the mean streets of a dirt-poor ghetto, or what has now been designated as "The Inner City." Although located a mere twenty road miles from the opulence of Bel Air, Beverly Hills, and Brentwood, in reality miles it might as well be a million. Whenever I mention the name of the area to friends, it always gets an instant visceral reaction.

First some definitions. As I said, all psychiatrists are doctors. We all graduated from medical school. We chose psychiatry as our area of specialization, just as others selected cardiology or surgery. And, like all medical specialists, we must finish a rigorous training program to perfect our craft.

While in training, a doctor works at only one hospital. The first year you are known as an "intern." For the next three years you are called a "resident" (aptly named). Collectively, all the hospitals' interns and residents are known as the "house staff." The physicians who supervise those in training are called "attendings." When an attending and his assigned interns and residents visit or discuss patients, this is called "rounds." When a housestaff member works all day, all night and all the next day this is known as being "on call."

Being on call doesn't mean you go home and only return for emergencies either. It means you stay in the hospital the entire day-night-and-day seeing to all the problems, large and small, that crop up in a busy county hospital: new admissions, discharges, sudden illnesses, ordering lab work, X rays, medicines, ER consultations, and patient evaluations for the walk-in triage area.

Enough of that. What of the story? The story of the year I spent as an intern at County General, The Bin. It's the story of a great many things, some of which I understand, some of which I don't and probably never will. On the surface, it's the story of one year in the making of a psychiatrist and as such is a story about doctors: what makes them tick, how they feel, why they do what they do. But, of course, it's a story about much, much more. It's a story about mental illness, about the mentally ill, about people who are mentally ill. It's a story about facing mental illness directly, person to person. It's a story about facing yourself.

It's more a process, really, than a story. A process that bears no artificial constraints of days, weeks, months, or years. It's the ongoing evolution of human beings caught in a storm of feelings, circumstance, and disease.

It's a process, this story, that ultimately, for me, came down to basic elements. Could I as one person assist another person in pain? Or more to the point, could I learn to connect with, to talk to and understand, really understand, another human being? It's been my privilege to have been a small part of this story, a privilege I pray I will never devalue or dishonor.

PSYCHWARD

ONE

SATAN'S FACE

I

JULY 1988

I WAS DRESSED in gray slacks, a white shirt, and the blue silk tie I'd been given the previous Christmas. My shoes were shined. My white laboratory coat was pressed and starched. I took a deep breath and slid my key into the locked door of Ward Three, the station to which I'd been assigned. I had a professional, confident smile on my face. Inside, I was terrified. It was eight A.M. I was thirty-eight years old. It was my first day as a psychiatrist-in-training.

Before turning the lock, I glanced through a small glass window in the metal door. With a start I dropped my keys. There was a face staring back at me. It was an angry face with steely, unwavering eyes. I tried to turn away but couldn't. It was those eyes. They were smoldering from the heat of some unseen fire burning behind them. The hair on the back of my neck stood up. A cold chill ran down my spine. It was the same feeling you get walking through a bad part of town when footsteps suddenly start up behind you. My pulse began to race. And still the man stared.

Then, as quickly as the young man had come, he was gone. A burly attendant was walking him back down the hall. It took me awhile to compose myself. Then I finally unlocked the door.

As I made my way down the tiled corridor, past the rows of small, three-bed dorm-type rooms in which the patients slept, by the common dayroom where a dozen people sat smoking and idly staring at a black-and-white television appended to a near wall, then into the cramped, glassed-in nursing station in which the ward staff was slowly accumulating to begin the day, I could not get that man's face out of my mind. I couldn't shake the feeling that I'd seen those eyes before.

"Who are you?" a middle-aged black woman dressed in nurse's white said looking me up and down as I stood in the corner of the nursing station.

"I'm Doctor Seager. Your new intern," I replied with a smile.

"Intern, huh?" The woman continued giving me the once-over. "You're too old," she said.

"I'm young at heart," I replied, trying to crack her icy stare.

"You're white," she said.

"I know that."

Then she shrugged. "Won't last a week," she sighed and turned away.

It had been ten years since I was first an intern, and after a decade of medical practice certain facts of training had slipped from my memory. But now everything was suddenly crystal clear again. In a teaching hospital an intern is low man on the totem pole, a sea slug in the evolution of a specialist. As I stood there in the busy nursing station, I felt I should grab a mop and do the floor.

After our brief encounter, the nurse—Elaine Givens, RN, her name tag read—retrieved a tray of small juice cups from the adjacent medication room and set them on the ledge of a Dutch-style door, the top half of which was open into the hallway.

Nurse Givens looked up and down the corridor then leaned her head out. "MEDICATION!" she suddenly shouted, and for the second time that morning I jumped back. It was like someone had fired a cannon. That voice would have brought drill sergeants to attention.

The patients on Ward Three may have been mentally ill but they weren't fools. When you're called like that you come. One by one, twenty people lined up for their morning medicine.

You have to understand something. Psychiatry, at least hospital psychiatry—life behind the locked doors where true mental illness lives—is just as foreign and frightening to most physicians as it is to the lay person. Only recently have psychiatric wards become a part of the average hospital, part of anywhere near the mainstream. For centuries the mentally ill were housed in dismal asylums or large state facilities as far from town as possible. Very few people, doctors included, ever visited there. Doctors, after all, are people, too, and the strange gut fear of mental illness affects them just as strongly as anyone, perhaps even more so. Medicine is, after all, a thinking profession and, as such, diseases of the mind, diseases of thinking, strike physicians at some very basic, rarely inspected core. It elicits instinctual, almost genetic fears. Until that morning, I had never seen a locked psychiatric unit. So I was not merely a casual observer watching those twenty people line up for medication: I was combatting some very scary images and emotions myself.

The whole process couldn't have taken more than ten minutes, but it had a profound effect on me. During that short medication ritual I realized that, despite all my credentials and experience, I knew little if anything about medicine and even less about myself. I could recite numbers and compose long lists of diseases. I knew a hundred drugs inside and out, but suddenly that seemed to pale in significance. At that moment, I realized I knew nothing about medicine because I knew nothing about people.

As the patients each appeared in turn at the window to receive and swallow the contents of their assigned juice cup, this gruff nurse with the jet-engine voice underwent a metamorphosis. She greeted each person by name, being certain to give due respect by using Mr. or Mrs. rather than a first name. She took a few moments to speak with everyone. "How are you feeling, Mr. Wilson?" "What's happening with your children, Mrs. Rogers?" "How about those Dodgers?" she said to an elderly black man who smiled but said nothing. She touched arms and squeezed hands and patted shoulders. Even the most severely ill people, those lost in some surreal inner world of madness, received the same warmth, the same touch, the same smile. It was an extraordinary example of simple human kindness.

Miss Givens had treated those twenty suffering souls like people. People to whom you could speak. People who deserved your respect. Those people weren't "feebs" or "loonies" or "crazies," they were just people. Like you and me. She hadn't joked. She hadn't ridiculed. She hadn't recoiled. She had spoken and touched.

Education, I suppose, is where you find it.

II

Dr. Rajib Singh was impeccably dressed in a gray suit and dark British regimental tie. His fifty-year-old face was tan and smooth. He wore a carefully manicured beard and a meticulously wrapped blue turban.

"Doctor Seager," he said in a brisk, Indian-tinged English clip. "Would you be so kind as to enlighten us on the major side effects of lithium carbonate and your understanding of the red blood cell membrane sodium pump?" It was morning rounds. Dr. James Patterson, a youngish, overweight black doctor with a slight southern drawl, the ward's chief resident, was seated to my left. Then came Dr. Singh at the head of the conference table. Miss Givens, an aide, another nurse, and Dr. Lamb, the staff psychologist, sat across from me. Dr. Lamb and Miss Givens were chatting quietly and smiling. Dr. Patterson was intent on a note he was writing in a patient's chart. As Dr. Singh spoke, however, all activity ceased and everyone stared at me. Suddenly the room was very warm.

"Pardon me?" I said, leaning forward in my chair, hoping desperately that I'd heard incorrectly.

"The major side effects of lithium, please," Singh repeated cooly. "And the RBC sodium pump."

"I'm new," I said with a nervous smile. I'd heard of lithium before but, as is the case with most non-psychiatrists, knew little about it, and what small amount of information I had managed to retain instantly vanished. So I just sat there smiling and sweating, hoping that if God ever chose to strike me dead it would be right then.

Dr. Singh said nothing for a moment. Then he fixed his gaze directly to mine. "You are a psychiatric intern, correct?" he said.

"Yes, sir," I replied weakly.

"I see," he said after another excruciating silence. "Perhaps tomorrow when you are not so 'new,' your memory will be a little more clear." Then he turned to Dr. Patterson. "You began our new patient, Mr. Jones, on Haldol yesterday," he said. "Be so kind as to inform the group concerning the proposed mechanism of action for the butyrophenone class of neuroleptics."

"Haldol is a high potency antipsychotic similar in strength to Prolixin," Patterson said without missing a beat, and for the next five minutes he detailed, in articulate fashion, the exact answer to Dr. Singh's question. He discussed the drug's history, its dosage range, what seemed like an endless stream of side effects (I lost count at fifteen), and all of the medicine's possible uses. He used phrases like "the dopamine hypothesis," "D_2 receptor blockade," "neuroleptic malignant syndrome" in a beautifully flowing stream of facts, figures, and theories about which I knew absolutely nothing. He might as well have been speaking Chinese. When he finished I could only stare in disbelief. I think my mouth actually dropped open. This was my second moment of revelation that morning.

What little exposure I had gleaned from my brief rotation in psychiatry during medical school had done nothing to prepare me for the complex, sophisticated world of neuroscience into which I had just entered. I had always pictured psychiatrists as bald men who sat around chatting. Now, suddenly, first question out of the gate, I had been asked to explain the intricate physiological pump system used to transport monovalent cations across cellular barriers.

Rounds lasted just over an hour. Mercifully, Dr. Singh spared me further agony, directing the remainder of his questions to others around the table. With the meeting at an end, as the staff slowly filed out of the room, Dr. Patterson, a knowing smile on his face, stood and patted me on the shoulder. "Wasn't what you expected, was it?" he said.

I could only shake my head.

"I had the same reaction," he went on. "We all did. You'll catch on quick. Don't worry."

At last I stood. My knees were none too steady. "I'd better," I replied. "I just hope I haven't screwed things up forever with Doctor Singh."

Patterson chuckled. "You mean the Mad Mahatma? Don't worry about him. He likes you. He asked a really tough question to the last intern." I smiled wanly.

"By the way," I said, catching Patterson at the door. "Why do I know that young white guy with the scary stare?" That face, those eyes had been on my mind all during rounds.

Patterson's face suddenly turned serious. "That's Ricky Myers," he said. "In the flesh."

"Didn't he kill some folks at a family picnic or something a few years back?" My memory was suddenly fresh as I recalled the nausea I'd felt while reading the newspaper account of those grisly murders.

"Stabbed eleven people," Patterson said quietly.

I felt that chill again. "What's he doing here?" I asked. "Shouldn't he be in prison or something?"

Patterson pulled out two chairs and we both sat back down. "Myers was declared insane at the trial," he said, leaning back a bit. "Then about six months ago, some half-assed shrink thought Ricky was well and the court released him from the state hospital. Last night he slashed two nine-year-old girls on their way home from school."

We were both silent for a moment. "Don't sweat it," Patterson said finally. "He'll only be your patient for a while. He's being transferred back to the state soon."

Sensing my acute uneasiness, Patterson leaned forward. "You've never seen a bad paranoid schiz before, have you?"

"Only on the news," I said. My mouth was dry.

"Don't ever forget the feeling you had when you first saw Myers," Patterson continued. "These people make your skin crawl for a reason. Remember Charlie Manson? Let me give you a few simple rules about dealing with these guys," he went on. "Treat them exactly like you would a strange dog in an alley. Never initiate a casual conversation. You don't know who they think you are. They may believe you're the devil. Never stare them in the eye. Never touch them. And above all, when they speak, you listen. If you're frightened, tell them so. Be firm, polite, and direct." Patterson spread his hands on the table. "And don't ever turn your back," he said slowly, his voice unwavering.

I thought for a minute, then nodded my head. I took Dr. Patterson's advice to heart and it served me in good stead. The majority of the staff seemed to do the same as well. There were a few, however, perhaps owing to the casualness that familiarity breeds, that did otherwise. It would prove to be an unfortunate mistake. It would cost one of them their lives.

After Patterson left I took a moment alone in the small conference room to collect my thoughts. I wasn't used to feeling frightened, stupid, and incompetent. It took awhile before I could show my face again in the nursing station. My spirits were buoyed, however, by the fact that now I was finally about to meet my patients. At last I would be in familiar territory. I had been an ER doctor for years. I'd interviewed thousands of patients. I thought my day was about to improve.

I chose the chart of Carl Williams first. Over the previous weeks I had laboriously written a ten-page outline culled from a number of texts on the structure and content of a thorough psychiatric interview. Before venturing onto the floor, I took a minute to review my notes one last time. I had rehearsed them a million times in my mind, like a graduation speech, but I felt one last glance couldn't hurt. I desperately wanted everything to go well.

At last I felt ready. I was prepared to delve into the far reaches of Carl Williams's past, have it revealed to me piece by piece and, from that, I would form a coherent structure of his inner workings and problems. I had reams of questions about childhood, parents, schooling, work, relationships, personal habits, emotions, medications, everything I could think of that would allow me to know, really know, Carl Williams. I had a blank pad of paper in my hands and two new pens in my pocket. I was armed to the teeth.

Carl Williams was a young man of twenty-four. He had unkempt blonde hair. His shirt was misbuttoned. As we walked from his room to my small ward office, he lost a slipper in the hallway but didn't seem to notice.

"Please sit down," I said, motioning to one of two utilitarian metal chairs on either side of a bare wooden desk. Carl Williams sat.

"Tell me," I said calmly, sitting in the other chair and clicking my pen. "What happened that you had to come to the hospital?" It was a thrilling moment. I was about to launch out into the sea of psychiatry.

Carl Williams smiled. "I'm an alien from the planet Zano," he replied.

I stared for a moment. "Pardon me?" I mumbled.

"Fuck you," he said and left the room.

I unclicked my pen, looked at my notes, and sighed. When I finally left the hospital late that night, the hubcaps were gone from my car.

TWO

NIGHT CALL

I

"CORNELIUS BROWN was brought in by the police on an involuntary hold," Dr. Amos Marks, a rail-thin young black doctor with a Van dyke moustache and close-cropped haircut, said wearily, checking his list of patients to be signed out to me and Dr. Manuel Lopez, a short, smiling Filipino, the senior resident with whom I would spend my first night on call. "Mr. Brown was found crawling down the center lane of the interstate. He was naked." Dr. Marks smiled. "The cops immediately recognized this as abnormal. They're sharp that way." He tapped his pencil on the small desk around which we were seated. His voice quickly regained its professional clip. "No psych history. Nystagmus on exam. It took seven of us to get him in restraints. I gave him Ativan and Haldol. He's sleeping now."

Dr. Lopez checked the first name off his list. "PCP?" he said.

"What else?" Marks replied.

"Next is Randell Richards, a thirty-year-old black male also brought in by the police," Marks went on, his face impassive. "He ran into a department store claiming a gorilla was chasing him. Then he went into the men's room and took a bath in the toilet. Long history of mental illness. Mother says he hasn't been taking his meds."

"No kidding," Lopez sighed.

"Chronic schiz undiff," Marks went on. "I restarted his Prolixin and began Cogentin."

Lopez and Marks both checked the second name off their lists. Then they broke into big smiles. "Bessie Thomas is back?" Lopez grinned.

"In all her glory," Marks replied. "She's an old bipolar," he said to me. "We've all taken care of her at one time or another. So will you."

"Bipolar?" I said uncomfortably. I'd never heard the word before.

"Manic-depressive," Marks said, looking quizzically at Lopez.

"I'm new," I replied, wondering how long that excuse would cover my ignorance. My stomach started to hurt.

"Does she think she's pregnant again?" Lopez asked.

"Of course," Marks replied.

"How many kids does this make now?" Lopez asked.

"According to her, four hundred," Marks said. "But who's counting?"

Lopez chuckled. "Who's she married to this time?" he asked.

"Prince Charles," Marks said, nodding his head. "I guess she divorced Michael Jackson."

Then Marks seemed to remember I was there and glanced at me with a look I couldn't read. It was either total pity or utter disdain. "Bipolars have delusions," he said.

"I didn't even know Michael Jackson was married," I said, and Marks smiled.

And so went sign-out rounds for night call. I'd only been on the ward three days and in the next twenty minutes twelve patients were turned over to Dr. Lopez and myself: A tiny, poorly dressed elderly woman who had wandered away from God knows where; a man who thought he was Elvis Presley; people talking to themselves; people hearing the voice of God; people who thought they were God; people so depressed they couldn't speak. And drug abusers who'd found themselves chewing grass on someone's lawn with urine-stained pants. Lopez and Marks flashed diagnoses and drug names back and forth like sword fighters. I tried to take everything down, but it was a losing battle. Finally, I just set my pen aside and listened. Then, his report at an end, Dr. Marks gave us a malevolent smile and stood to leave. "They're all yours," he said. "Good luck."

I felt far from confident for many reasons. One was especially troubling. In the three days I'd worked on the ward I'd watched my patients line up for medication every morning and afternoon, and one by one down a small, plastic cup of Sunkist fruit juice. I thought the pharmacy had a special way of dissolving the medication inside. It seemed reasonable enough. After all, that way no one could "cheek" his pills and not receive the proper dose. How they sealed the foil back on top I hadn't a clue.

That made it all the more disconcerting when, upon arriving in PES—Psychiatric Emergency Service, "service" being a medical term for the emergency ward itself—for my call, I saw the nurses and orderlies talking quietly in the lounge, all sipping little cups of Sunkist juice.

So, there I stood, watching Dr. Marks close that big metal door behind him. A man was screaming, "Mother, I'm coming!" in the background. An orderly had opened a closet and was counting his stock of sturdy leather restraints. There was the odd shout and groan coming from the rooms behind me. Finally, a three-hundred-pound woman wearing a bedsheet wrapped garrishly around her body and with a brassiere on her head passed by. "Prince Charles has a big dick," she said and then laughed hysterically.

I could only sigh. I was locked inside with these people. We were deep in the heart of a miserable ghetto. It was getting dark outside. And my staff was all taking heavy medication. It was going to be a long night.

Early the following morning a nurse noticed me staring intently as she prepared the day's first round of medicines. "The pills go in a small cup on the side," she said without looking up. "It's a common mistake."

II

To understand the mentally ill and their care, as I was learning to do, it's necessary to be clear on a few basic points. In general, society doesn't care anything about the mentally ill, never has, never will. The insane behave erratically, they don't vote, and they don't pay taxes. People simply don't want them around. At best, they are ignored, at worst, abused.

Our treatment of the mad has, with few exceptions, remained remarkably constant over the centuries. It boils down to this: The mentally ill act strangely, so we torment them. Whether we believed they were possessed by demons, cursed by God, or, as the more contemporary thinking goes, they suffer from inherited neurochemical disorders, their lot has historically remained pretty much the same.

When millenia of burnings and torture didn't rid us of them, we built large warehouse-style institutions to keep them out of our hair. This worked for a while; then attorneys got involved and we let everyone out again. We called it "deinstitutionalization." We said we were protecting their civil rights. Besides, it was cheaper than feeding them all.

And so, their rights intact, the mentally ill are once again back in the community, back where they came from, back among the people who didn't want them in the first place. We have, however, at least given them new names. Now the insane are known as "the homeless" or "bag ladies" or, more generically, just "street people."

Of course, we are more sophisticated and civilized than our medieval forefathers. We no longer let the insane suffer in the name of God—that would be foolish. Now they suffer in the name of legal liberty. And we have absolved the clergy from performing our dirty work. In the spirit of free enterprise, we contract out the job. The mentally ill are now plundered and harassed by gangs of urban street thugs and other human vultures. I recently read where two "transients" were found decapitated in a dumpster. Each had a prescription bottle of Thorazine in his pocket.

That is the debit side. To our credit, the mentally ill are probably eating better than they did previously. I know for a fact that the regular collection of ragged people who frequent the large throw-away bins behind the supermarkets in my neighborhood often find perfectly good fruits and vegetables.

When the chronically mentally ill run afoul of the law, they are brought to County General, The Bin. There they see me or others like me. We give them medication, food, and a bed to sleep in for a while. Then we have to release them. It's the law. And an entire array of legal and hospital personnel exist merely to be certain that the law is enforced. Our social workers refer them to board-and-care homes that in many ways resemble, in scaled-down form, the very institutions from which they were turned out. From there they wander back to the street. Then, if they don't die from the cold or an untreated infection or get lit on fire, they will find their way back to The Bin and the whole process begins again. And so it goes.

And don't think this is strictly a Los Angeles problem, because it's not. We are an egalitarian society: The misery is equally shared everywhere. There are tattered people talking to the air from coast to coast. It's not strictly a big city concern either. I know for a fact there is a busy medical clinic for the homeless in Ogden, Utah.

I will grant some regional differences in the mentally ill, however. When one of our former patients is found dead in his piano-crate home, he probably has a better tan than the corpses from other areas.

III

I met Martin Braga that first night on call. Martin was not chronically mentally ill. He had, as far as I knew, never lived in a board-and-care home or selected his dinner from a garbage can. At least not yet, that is. Dr. Lopez was busy doing a consultation in the main hospital ER, so I was by myself in the triage station, the small lobby-like area adjacent to the locked wards where people could walk in off the street and talk to a psychiatrist. Triage means "sorting out." It's where the decision is made to hospitalize or not. From there patients to be admitted go downstairs one floor to the PES, a locked holding area, until their beds are ready up on the wards. At night the triage area and PES are manned by the intern and resident on call. Dr. Lopez and I had seen a number of patients together that evening. Martin Braga was the first I saw alone.

The automatic sliding doors opened and a family walked in. A middle-aged Hispanic woman and her husband were obviously upset. You could tell she had been crying. Three young men were with them, apparently their sons. The two older boys, tall and tan, were bookending their younger brother between them. The third son, smaller than the other two, was dressed in a dirty shirt and wrinkled pants. He seemed preoccupied with his own thoughts, hardly aware, it appeared, of where he was or what was happening. Occasionally he would mutter something to himself and laugh. This was Martin Braga.

After Martin's parents had completed the necessary paperwork, I took them all into our small interview room. Martin and his parents sat on a battered couch in front of my bare metal desk. His two brothers took seats on folding chairs to the side. Everyone, most of all myself, was tense and apprehensive. Our initial conversation was stilted and overly proper. Then a critical point was reached and the flood gates broke. Suddenly, the entire family wanted to talk at once, except for Martin who had been staring at me in silence since we'd entered the room. But it wasn't a normal stare. He was looking at me but he didn't seem to be seeing me. His eyes were lifeless, like those of a dead man. All the while Martin's parents spoke I kept returning to those eyes. They never flickered once.

For the next twenty minutes Martin's parents told me a story that would, regrettably, become an all-too-familiar one over the next year. They said that Martin had been a good son, a college student with many friends and a bright future. Then, suddenly, everything changed. They told of Martin slowly just drifting away, gradually spending more and more time alone in his room, finally isolating himself from everyone completely. They said he'd begun to speak of laser beams and the CIA. He said he was receiving messages from outer space. He believed his food was poisoned.

I tried to imagine the scenes that must have occurred in the Braga home over the past few months. I couldn't begin to comprehend the despair and frustration these poor people must have felt as they watched their son and brother deteriorate right before their eyes.

"Why did you wait so long to get help?" I said at last.

Mrs. Braga began to weep quietly. I felt like kicking myself. "I'm sorry," I blurted instantly. "I didn't mean . . ."

"That's okay, Doctor," Mr. Braga said with a sad smile. "We know we should have come in earlier. We realized Martin was very ill. We just prayed that somehow it would all go away. That it wouldn't be the same."

"The same?" I asked.

Mr. Braga sighed. "My wife's brother had this happen to him too," he said slowly. "He's been in and out of mental hospitals most of his life. We were hoping against hope."

For the next minute everyone in the room sat in silence. All except Martin, that is. Martin suddenly began mumbling in a low, steady voice. "Jesus is the devil. Jesus is the devil," he said over and over again.

I admitted Martin Braga to the hospital that night. He was in the middle of his first schizophrenic break. It was the beginning of a long road for both of us. Over the coming months Martin Braga would teach me more about mental illness than I could have learned from a dozen textbooks. He would teach me more about suffering and compassion than I had thought possible. I would come to know Martin Braga as well as I had ever known anyone. For me, Martin Braga turned on the light.

IV

All in all, that first night on call was nothing if not interesting. I got to see my first PCP overdose, a nineteen-year-old boy who'd cut off the end of his left thumb thinking it was the head of a snake. I admitted people who were hearing voices, sedated those in a wired panic from too much cocaine, and referred out an army of tired and hungry souls who weren't mentally ill but had come to the hospital simply because there was nowhere else to go. Then, just before dawn, I saw my final two patients. And for one of them, Mrs. Bennett, I took my first stab at psychotherapy.

There is an aphorism in psychiatry that says simply: "Talking helps." As Dr. Lopez explained, patients can derive a great deal of benefit from just having someone listen to them. So when Mrs. Bennett sat down and began to speak, I listened. As this depressed forty-five-year-old black woman told of the grief she'd suffered after her only son had been killed in a gang shooting, I listened. When she spoke of her husband leaving her for a younger woman, I listened. When she painfully recounted the physical and sexual abuse she'd suffered as a child, I listened.

The hour passed quickly. When our time was up, I realized I had barely spoken. I hadn't offered Mrs. Bennett any advice or insight. When she'd cried, I'd touched her arm. And then listened some more. I hadn't given her quick suggestions or reached for my prescription pad. I hadn't done any of the things I'd thought being a doctor was all about.

But something happened during that hour, something good. As Mrs. Bennett stood to leave, she actually smiled. She took my hand in hers and said, "Thank you." Suddenly there was a small tear in both our eyes.

I made Mrs. Bennett an appointment with our outpatient clinic and bade her goodbye. As I watched her walk out the door back into the night, I was overcome with a wonderful feeling. I thought I'd helped.

Soon after that I saw my last patient, Mr. Thompson, or, as he would come to be known, Harry Houdini. Barely an hour after I first saw Mr. Thompson and had sent him downstairs, I lost him. Or he disappeared. Or something. Somehow the man just vanished.

Mr. Thompson, a thin black man of fifty with rags on his back and fire in his eyes, was brought in by the police who'd placed him on an involuntary seventy-two-hour hold. In California, policemen can do this. So can psychiatrists. If we believe you are a danger to yourself, a danger to others, or "gravely disabled," i.e., unable to provide for your own food, clothing, and shelter, we can keep you in a psychiatric hospital against your will. If, after those three days are up, you still meet the same criteria, we can keep you for two weeks more.

All things considered, in this day and age, that is pretty powerful stuff. It's nothing, of course, like the open-ended commitment powers of old, but fairly heady business nonetheless. At least that's how I was thinking about it back then. It would take me awhile to learn that in the world of curing mental illness, seventeen days is a Band-Aid at best.

I had our security people escort Mr. Thompson downstairs. He was in handcuffs and, although he couldn't have weighed more than a hundred and thirty pounds holding two bricks, he put up quite a struggle. It took four big guards to wrestle him into the elevator and two more to finally get him strapped to a bed.

The paperwork left by the police said Mr. Thompson had become agitated at a local market. They said he'd attacked two elderly patrons with a stick.

I followed Mr. Thompson downstairs to the PES, our locked emergency holding area, where I gave him an injection of Haldol and Ativan, a combination of major tranquilizer and fast-acting Valium, and inside of twenty minutes he was quiet. I didn't think much more about him until the nurse who'd gone in to release him from restraints came running back down the hall.

"He's gone," she said simply.

"I don't understand," I replied, looking up from a chart.

The nurse motioned me over and we made for Mr. Thompson's room. The door was still locked. Through a small window I could see his bed. There were the four leather restraints, each still securely tied to the metal bed frame. But there was no Mr. Thompson.

Hurriedly the nurse unlocked the door and we rushed inside. We checked the bathroom. We checked under the bed. We checked the bathroom again. Then we called upstairs for help and everyone searched the entire ward. We looked in every bathroom and under every bed. When we began opening cabinet doors I knew we were licked.

Slowly, all the nurses and security people gathered back in the main hallway. After a few moments of silence, a guard looked back into Mr. Thompson's room. "That's odd," he said finally.

For the next hour security men scoured the hospital grounds. We called in a missing-person report to the police, somewhat sheepishly I must admit. But nothing turned up. No Mr. Thompson.

Then it was morning and Dr. Marks was back. He came in smiling. That soon changed. Quickly, Dr. Lopez and I gave him a rundown on the patients we'd admitted overnight. I saved Mr. Thompson for last. "We put him in restraints," I said. "Then he disappeared."

Dr. Marks only sighed and pinched the bridge of his nose.

After leaving the PES, Dr. Lopez suggested we get something to eat before starting the day. I shook my head. "He'll turn up," Dr. Lopez said finally. "He has to, doesn't he?"

THREE

ANITA AND BONES

I

ANITA ASHWIN looked like a porcelain doll. Or something from a picture out of the Arabian Nights. She was bright, witty, and sincere. She had the serene smile of a contented angel. Anita was from Bangalore, India, where she'd taken her medical degree.

Anita was classified as a "foreign medical graduate," or FMG for short. I had been trained at a large eastern medical school and, unfortunately, had many of the same stereotypic ideas about FMGs as did the majority of my American colleagues. The consensus was that they were poorly trained (after all they hadn't gone to American schools), that they couldn't speak English very well and, as such, were perforce not as intelligent as the rest of us. Most American residents smugly maintain these beliefs. That is, until they meet some FMGs.

The foreign medical graduates in our program were, with few exceptions, intelligent, articulate, good doctors. This was especially true of Anita Ashwin. She'd been a board-certified internist back home, but owing to an incredible amount of bureaucratic bias and baloney, was unable to find a medicine training slot in this country.

She had opted for psychiatry instead. As Anita said, psychiatry positions are easier for FMGs to get. Most American training hospitals are located in the decaying hearts of large cities and this, for many reasons, is where most of the mentally ill are as well. Poverty and insanity is not an attractive combination for most American doctors. "Since you're not interested in caring for these people," Anita said to me one afternoon, "it's left to us."

Anita was a second-year psychiatric resident who came to Ward Three at the beginning of August, my second month, replacing Dr. Patterson from whom I'd learned a great deal. Dr. Patterson had advised me on the correct medication regimens for my patients, especially Martin Braga, whose voices had now stopped. He'd shown me the ropes on the inpatient ward, who to ask for what, what numbers to call to get things done, which people to avoid and which to approach. He taught me to push all the right buttons. It was invaluable information. Dr. Patterson had given me the nuts and bolts of psychiatry. From Dr. Ashwin I would learn its heart and soul.

Anita Ashwin didn't teach me the psychiatry of medicines, neuro-chemicals, or humoral receptors: I could get that from my reading. She gave me the key to intrapersonal connection. She taught me how to relate to the mentally ill. She taught me how to see the situation from their point of view. And she did it with one word.

"Empathy," she said softly, holding an index finger in the air for emphasis.

"Empathy?" I replied somewhat confused. It was after rounds and Dr. Singh had grilled me again. I just wasn't getting enough information from my patients. Dr. Ashwin had noticed my frustration and taken me aside into a quiet room.

"Be concerned about your patients," she said. "Not about their disease but about them as people. That's the most important lesson I can teach you. Most people are mistaken about psychiatry, and I suspect at this point you are, too. The secret is not in making incisive

38

interpretations and erudite analysis. These things are important, of course, but not fundamental. Empathy is." She smiled at me and went on. "Think what it must be like to be mentally ill. You're always in people's way, always bothering someone, always getting in everybody's hair for reasons that you can't understand. Imagine the average person's reaction to the things our patients say and do. Then imagine what a relief it must be to have someone just sit and listen. To talk to you. To be concerned about you. Someone who doesn't tell you to go away or recoil in fright. This is the greatest gift you can give your patients, the gift of yourself, your time, your understanding. If they like and trust you, they will give you all the facts you need.

"It is not the patient's job," she continued, "to adjust to your reality. It's your job to relate to his. Patients are like trains moving along on their own track at their own speed. If you get in the way, only disaster will result. You must alter your pace, your direction and somewhere, somehow, climb on board." Again she smiled that calm smile. "It's a journey that you will find very rewarding. I guarantee it."

As you might gather I liked Anita Ashwin a great deal and respected her even more. She was an insightful and genuinely caring person. Unfortunately, it was these very qualities that got her into trouble.

Anita tried to connect with everyone, to listen to everyone, to help everyone no matter how difficult or challenging the case. If there was a patient no one else wanted, she would always volunteer her services. In our part of town there was one particular group of people nobody cared to handle. The stakes were just too high. So, naturally, it was to them that Dr. Ashwin, the diminutive Indian woman, naturally gravitated. She developed a special affinity for the problems of gang members.

I had visited County General fifteen years before coming there as a psychiatric resident. I was different then. The place was different then. Lots of things were different then. This was back before they called it The Bin. Back before the apathy. Back before the violence and ugliness. Back before The Beast arrived. Back before cocaine.

In every American ghetto cocaine is big business. It's really the only business. And everywhere—New York, Miami, Chicago, Phoenix, etc.—a new set of entrepreneurs has arisen to handle the myriad details of its distribution. Be they black, white, Asian or Latino, marketing cocaine is what gangs do. They are the drug network. They do the bloodletting. They haul in the rock and pack out the bodies. They are a nation and law unto themselves. They have the structure and purpose that the ghetto lacks. They also have guns and money. This is a bad combination.

Some gang members also use cocaine. Cocaine can make you act crazy. That's how we get involved in all this. "If I can just save one of them," Dr. Ashwin said to me once, "somehow break the cycle of drugs and violence, then it will all be worth it."

A week after she'd come to Ward Three, Dr. Ashwin introduced me to one of her angry young men. He had a colored kerchief on his head and stone in his heart. His name was Reggie, but everyone called him "Bones." Bones was a "Blue." The Blues were the newest and fastest growing of our inner-city gangs. The Blues fought with the Greens, a larger, more established gang. Each group had their own style of dress and speech. Each had their own distinctive graffiti. The Blues murdered with AK-47s. The Greens used Uzis.

I often wondered if Dr. Ashwin had a clear idea about what was really going on, what she was getting herself into. She was from India. She wore a sari. She spoke of connecting and empathy. I was worried.

Anita got a call from Bones a few days after I'd met him. It took her awhile to calm him down. "I'll see you at four," she said finally and hung up. Catching my nervous look she gave me one of her patented smiles. It did have a way of soothing people. Maybe I'm all wrong about this, I thought. I was new to the business, after all. Besides, I had enough problems of my own. I had patients to see.

II

It had been just over a month since I'd made my first nervous entry onto Ward Three. I wouldn't say that I'd settled in, but things were definitely more familiar. I was still a little anxious now and then, but fortunately I had Dr. Ashwin with me.

I saw my four patients for thirty minutes each during the afternoons. I always started with Ricky Myers, the mass murderer. That way things could only improve the rest of the day. Somehow Myers's transfer to the state facility had gotten snagged. So, until that red tape got untangled, he was mine.

Even on heavy doses of medication, Ricky Myers was a distinctly frightening individual. No amount of drug, it seemed, could dim that terrifying glint in his eye. He still made my spine freeze. I followed two of Dr. Patterson's rules whenever I spoke with him. I always kept the door open and never let him get between me and a quick escape route. My sessions with Myers were short and shorter, depending on my own anxiety level that day. And today's was no different. Do you need anything? How are you sleeping? Are you still hearing voices? Thank you very much. Goodbye.

I know he could sense my fear. It was thick as fog. The man made my face twitch. I thought perhaps one day I might overcome my insecurities and be able to deal effectively with people like Ricky Myers. But somehow I doubted it.

I took some comfort in the fact that I wasn't the only person bothered by Ricky Myers. The other patients and most of the staff seemed just as frightened of him as I was. The nurses stepped lively whenever their duties took them into Myers's room. And the other patients gave him a wide, nervous berth when he made an infrequent foray into the hallway. It was like he was radioactive. You couldn't see it. You couldn't hear it. You simply knew that distance was the only thing you wanted between yourself and Ricky Myers.

Myers was the only patient on the ward with a room to himself. This hadn't been a conscious plan on the staff's part. I don't recall it ever being actually discussed. It was just the natural thing to do. Our fear of the man was so great that it didn't need verbal expression. We just assumed no one would want to live with Ricky Myers, to get to know him, much less close their eyes in his presence.

Dr. Singh alone didn't seem to share in the dread of Myers. Or if he did, he didn't show it. He always greeted Ricky when they passed and occasionally stopped to chat for a moment. He even made Myers smile once. I had to admire Dr. Singh. I imagined his aplomb stemmed from years of psychiatric experience. That the man could probably handle anything. I hoped I would be like that some day.

Carl Williams was more talkative now, but he was still Carl Williams. He no longer claimed to be an alien from the planet Zano, however; now he was a Klingon. He often spoke of capturing Captain Kirk. He said he had an elaborate plan to destroy the *Enterprise*. He only smiled when anyone asked about it.

Carl Williams was what was once called a "hebephrenic" or "silly" schizophrenic. He spent a good deal of time gazing into mirrors. He frequently assumed odd postures. He always looked as if he'd just remembered a particularly funny joke. I liked Carl Williams a lot. In his infrequent semi-lucid moments he spoke of having gone to college and about an old girlfriend. But then he also said his psychology professor had been Sigmund Freud and that his father was Harry Truman, so who knew?

When I spoke with Carl that afternoon, he was in excellent spirits.

He said his plan for Kirk and the *Enterprise* was at last complete. "Would you care to share it?" I asked.

"It involves Zirconite and droids from the moons of Magyar," he said proudly. "But, of course, you knew that."

"I'd always suspected," I said with a nod. "But I wasn't sure."

"Not a word to Kirk and the men," Carl whispered. Then he shook my hand and left. Walking back down the hall he laughed out loud.

Third on my list was Minnie Osbourne, a frail black twig of a woman with a smile as wide as the Mississippi Delta where she'd lived most of her eighty-three years. Her face was still unlined. Her eyes twinkled like dark stars.

Minnie had spent her life doing domestic work for wealthy white families around New Orleans. She'd raised six children, two of whom had gone on to college. Her oldest son, she claimed, was an attorney in New York City. She said her husband died during World War II fighting in Italy. Minnie could not recall why she had left the South.

Minnie wasn't mentally ill in the traditional sense of the word. She'd lived a long and productive life. A life that still gave no sign of losing any of its intensity or verve. She had, unfortunately, been stricken with a modern form of brain failure. Minnie had Alzheimer's disease.

Minnie had been found wandering in a vacant lot. She could not give an address or phone number. She couldn't remember the name of anyone she knew in the city. No one had reported her missing. So the police brought her to County General. They dumped her in The Bin.

Minnie could recount down to the finest detail what dress she'd worn, the exact scent of the azaleas, the faces of her gentlemen callers—all the events of her colorful and fascinating girlhood. She told me stories of crawdad hunting and picnics and of helping to serve for grand balls in the homes of her rich employers.

She could paint an exact picture of the family's small home outside

New Orleans, and describe exactly her feelings about being black in the South during the twenties and thirties. Unfortunately, she couldn't remember much else. That's the way Alzheimer's works. It unravels your life in reverse. It picks apart your mental foundation brick by brick, starting with today and working backward. Eventually, if left to its own devices, Alzheimer's will turn a person into an adult fetus. The thought is profoundly appalling.

Minnie not only had Alzheimer's, she was also nearly blind. Her eyes had begun to fail a few years back; she could not recall exactly when, and now the light was almost gone. This was a very real problem. There are tens of thousands of people with Alzheimer's disease residing in nursing homes. With Minnie being blind, however, and with no income, we couldn't find a single place willing to take her. "Too much trouble," they said routinely. So Minnie had taken up residence at County General.

Minnie and I spent many pleasant afternoon sessions talking about the old days and about her one, overriding passion—politics. "Franklin Delano Roosevelt," she said proudly. "He was my man. Voted for him four times. Would do it again, too, if I had the chance. The finest president we've had before or since." Minnie's voice, usually thin with a tremolo shake, became firm and full whenever she spoke of FDR. "He had a feel for the common man," she said. She told me how she'd once walked twenty miles just to see his train pass by.

Minnie was a kind, sweet woman and I loved her dearly. When we finally tracked down her son, the attorney in New York City, he said that placing his mother in a nursing home was fine with him but that he was too busy to come out and help with the arrangements. "Doesn't social security cover that?" he replied when we inquired about finances. Then he said he had to run. After that his office refused all our calls.

Finally I got to Martin Braga. It was three o'clock. Martin had been

44

on Haldol, a drug similar in effect to Thorazine, for a month now. The voices had stopped. He was no longer mumbling about Jesus and Satan. His clothing and hair were in reasonable order. Yet, something was still very wrong with Martin. I knew it and, unfortunately, so did he.

Martin took a seat across from me in my office. He looked ill at ease and slightly confused, as if negotiating a chair was a difficult experience for him. As if, somehow, chairs didn't feel like he thought they were supposed to feel.

It had taken some very awkward sessions before I got through to Martin even a little. Initially, while he was still acutely psychotic, before the Haldol took hold, there wasn't anything between us that could even remotely be considered conversation. Basically, Martin rambled and I nodded. Slowly, however, a person began to come through. Slowly, some trust and warmth began to emerge. Gradually we began to talk.

"How are you feeling today, Martin?" I asked. It was my standard opening.

But today I didn't get the standard reply. Today he didn't just say, "Fine." Today his lower lip began to tremble as did his hands.

"Is something frightening you?" I asked.

"You wanted to know how I felt," Martin said finally. "What did you mean?"

I was taken aback slightly. "I mean are you sad, happy, angry?" I answered. "How do you feel inside?"

Martin's shoulders dropped. "I think I know why you're asking the question," he said haltingly. "But somehow I just can't conjure up an answer. I know I used to feel things. But now, it's like I'm hollow or numb. Completely empty."

I didn't reply. After a moment, Martin continued. "It's as if we are talking across a great divide, like I'm looking at you from the wrong

45

end of binoculars. I know I could physically reach out and touch you. But I can't get a sense of you as a person. Everything is so cold and unreal."

Martin's voice had a slight monotone drone to it. The words were coming out in the correct order, but there was no inflection to them, no up and down, no pauses. It was like they were coming in over a teletype. "Sometimes I think I'm the only person left in the world," Martin continued. "The only person in the entire universe. It's like I'm floating alone out in a huge, hopeless black void. That no matter how hard I search or how long I float, I will never see another living human being again."

"You know I'm here for you," I said reassuringly. "And so is the rest of the staff."

"I appreciate that," Martin went on. "But then the void overwhelms me and it just doesn't matter. I can't explain it. Nothing seems to matter any more."

"Have the voices come back?" I asked.

Martin let out a semblance of a laugh. "I must be crazy to have heard voices," he said. "That's what happened to me, isn't it? I went crazy."

Now my words wouldn't come. "You . . . you had a . . ." I fumbled. Fortunately, Martin began to speak again.

"Schizophrenics hear voices, right?" Martin went on. "My uncle is schizophrenic. Is that what happened to me?" he asked. "Did I come down with schizophrenia?"

I didn't know what else to say. "Yes," I replied simply.

Martin's voice dropped in tone a bit and was suddenly touched with something close to emotion. "That's what I thought," he said.

I was immediately overwhelmed by the physician's instinct to offer some kind of hope. I began to speak rapidly. "It's not as bad as you might think," I said. "Many schizophrenics do very well. There are medications to control the voices and good treatment facilities here at the hospital. We can . . .” Then I noticed Martin wasn't listening any more. His face was impassive, his eyes dull and unfocused. I knew I was losing him to the void.

“Could I go back to my room now?” Martin said quietly.

I walked with Martin down the hall and opened the door to his room. He shuffled in, sat on the edge of his bed, and began staring blankly out the window. Martin stared out the window a lot. As I turned to go I had an ache in the pit of my stomach.

It was after four when I got back to the nursing station. I took my charts, found a quiet corner, and began to write my daily notes. I had just begun when I heard a strange string of popping noises in the distance. It sounded like firecrackers. Then there was a frantic voice over the hospital intercom paging all available security help to the triage area at once.

Suddenly I felt like I'd been struck with a cattle prod. “God, no!” I shouted and bolted for the door. Anita Ashwin had been seeing Bones in triage since four.

I pounded down the hall as fast as I could run. I dared not think the worst but the sound of that *pop-pop-pop* kept echoing in my ears.

Ahead of me two attendants burst through the door into triage. I clamored and skidded behind them. My head was throbbing and my lungs ached.

Then everything stopped. There wasn't a sound. No one was moving. Behind the front desk the clerk had one hand covering her mouth. There were fifteen people all standing frozen, like statues, all encircling the open door to the small interview room. Between their feet a tiny rivulet of bright red blood was slowly winding along the white tile. Gradually gaining speed, it meandered out into the center of the floor and began to form a small, round pool.

FOUR

LET THEM EAT CAKE

I

YOU NEVER GET used to it. I know. As a trauma doctor I'd dealt
with violent death hundreds of times before and it's always the same.
There is the initial wave of shock, of course, but with repetition this
tends to pass quickly. Then comes the numbness. The wave of nausea. But these things don't stick, either. What stays glued to your
memory, oddly enough, is the smell. The smell of fresh warm blood
spilled from ripped body parts. It's so faint and distinct an aroma that,
at first, you don't even realize it's there. You may not be aware of it for
a few hours or a few days even. But it always catches up with you.
Usually later when things are quiet and your mind drifts. It isn't a
smell you appreciate with your nose. It's a brain smell. A smell that
goes straight to some deep primitive center of your cortex. It's a
profoundly disquieting moment when the reality of that smell finally
hits. It's a feeling you can never quite shake.

I smelled that smell again when I slowly walked through the
stunned crowd and stood in front of the doorway to our small triage
interview room. Blood was everywhere. It looked as if a red volcano

49

had erupted. Mixed with the crimson splatters were tiny glinting gray pieces of human brain tissue.

To my right, Bones was splayed over the back of the couch in front of Dr. Ashwin's desk, his arms and legs frozen in a final, desperate tangle. Most of the blood running on the floor was coming from two cantaloupe-sized holes in his body; one directly in the center of his chest where his heart had been, the other had blown away his left hip. The rest of the blood was dripping from his head or at least what was left of his head. Everything from the nose up was gone.

Then to my left I saw Dr. Ashwin. Through a million red splotches that covered her face, she seemed to be staring at me. Her hands were on top of the desk. She was still holding her notebook. She looked exactly like what she was. Someone who'd been unexpectedly interrupted by a commotion at the door and was turning to speak.

Miraculously, she didn't seem to be hit. All the blood belonged to Bones. I was so relieved my knees almost buckled. I called Anita's name but it was lost in a sudden din of paramedics and policemen behind me. I hurriedly stepped aside as shouting people poured into the room in droves. The entire triage area was in instant pandemonium. The confusion began to overwhelm me. I knew if I didn't sit down I would fall.

I picked my way back through the excited throng and unlocked the door to Ward Three. Somehow I made it to the nursing station and collapsed into a chair. I can't remember what I thought about or what I was feeling. But I know I sat a very long time. When I finally stood to leave, the ward staff had all returned. When I looked out into triage again, it was empty save one lone man idly swiping at the floor with a mop and rinsing off the dusky water in a bucket.

Something else unusual about violent death is how quickly it's forgotten, how soon things return to normal. At least on the surface. By nightfall the police had swept the interview room for evidence, prying thirteen assault rifle shells from the walls and sealing them in

individually numbered plastic bags that were placed with other similar bags containing bits of hair and shreds of bloody cloth. The floor
was white again in no time. Statements from witnesses took a bit
longer. By midnight, however, everything was up and running again.
The waiting room was full, the desk clerk was typing rhythmically,
and in the small interview room Dr. Patterson, who'd been transferred
to Ward One when Anita arrived and was on call with me that
evening, sat across from a patient seated on the couch. His hands
were folded on top of the desk. He was holding a small notebook.

Bones was taken to the morgue. Dr. Ashwin went to the main
hospital ER across the street. Dr. Maxwell, the chairman of psychiatry, attended her. She was sedated and sent home. The next morning,
understandably, Anita was not at work. Nor for the next three days
after that. When she hadn't returned in a week, I began to get
frightened. I couldn't forget her eyes as she'd stared toward me in the
doorway. They were eyes that had watched a nightmare come true. I
was worried we might never see Dr. Ashwin again.

In the ghetto, a black man murdering another black man, even in a
hospital interview room, doesn't rouse much interest. There were no
TV cameras at the hospital the night Bones was killed. No reporters
came to get the "exclusive." For three days I searched the paper
looking for news. Finally I found a two-inch column on page seventeen of the city section. "Man Shot at Local Hospital" the small
headline read. The page-one story was about a Santa Monica attorney
who raised roses.

II

It was toward the end of August when we got the news. Things were
running fairly smoothly on Ward Three. Dr. Alice Lincoln, a no-

nonsense young black woman, was filling in for Anita Ashwin who had requested and received an unlimited leave of absence. Dr. Lincoln and I got along well, but I still missed Anita. I'd tried phoning her often but could only get an answering machine. I left messages, none of which were ever returned.

As always, I had a steady stream of patients in and out of the ward. With only seventeen days total allowed for involuntary commitment, there wasn't much real healing going on. We were like mechanics at a pit stop. We slapped a patch over the leak and got people back on the road.

I still had my core of four patients, Ricky Myers, Minnie Osbourne, Carl Williams, and Martin Braga, all of whom had either signed in voluntarily or had nowhere else they could or were allowed to go. And finally there was Mr. Thompson, the disappearing man. It had been weeks now and there was still no sign of him. The PES staff did note, however, that for the past while they had been consistently short in their count of patient dinner trays at the end of each evening shift.

And, strangely, there were a growing number of reports from different hospital departments of missing equipment. The nurses on Ward Two said their sheet and towel supplies were low. Miss Givens noticed an end table was missing from the nursing office. One morning, Dr. Maxwell came to work and found all the pictures gone from his consultation room walls. There were others as well, but the capper came from Ward One: They called security one day because someone had stolen an entire bed.

Anyway, the big news was this: The county, through whom all our mental health funding flowed, had experienced an unexpected shortfall in revenue. Corners, they said, would have to be cut. And, like pack animals responding to instinct, they instantly turned on their weakest member. The proposal was to slash our already pitiful budget in half. Apparently they didn't expect much reaction. Mental health money had been cut routinely over the years and, excepting larger crowds at supermarket trash bins, nothing much had come of it. This time, however, we vowed that things would be different. Enough was enough. We decided to mobilize. We decided to answer back in a language the board of supervisors would understand. We organized a voter registration drive.

Our target was Marvin "Big Daddy" Benson.

Benson, a large, jowly man of sixty and thirty-year member of the county board, had first been elected from our district back before the "demographics" changed, i.e., back before all the white people fled and all the black people moved in. But he had a firmly entrenched and highly efficent political machine behind him and, over the years, had been consistently re-elected.

Benson, everyone agreed, had always served his constituents well; at least he'd served well those constituents that mattered. He hadn't seemed to care much, however, for our local army of garbage bin eaters. But, truthfully, no one else had, either. Big Daddy was the main thrust behind the proposed budget cuts. He wanted money for a new freeway. He was up for another vote in November. We were determined to get his attention.

A history of mental illness is not an exclusionary criterion for voting. The mentally ill tend not to vote, however, because it takes an organized effort and organization is not their long suit. It also takes some degree of commitment to the system. For most of our patients, however, the system was strictly the means by which society exerted its profound indifference upon them. We knew we were facing an uphill battle.

Win or lose, our fledgling political effort had at least one positive result and it appeared almost immediately. The moment I mentioned our plan to Minnie Osbourne, the diminutive, elderly black woman, her face lit like a lamp. "Grassroots organization is the key," she said, becoming more excited by the minute. "That's what worked for

FDR. Four times he was elected president because he never lost touch with the people."

"Thank you, Minnie, but I think . . ." I said and was promptly cut off.

"Have you contacted the families?" Minnie continued, oblivious to my interruption. "Remember, every patient has parents, brothers, sisters, aunts, uncles, and cousins. They're all voters, too. Have you called the media?" she said directly to me.

"Well, no, not yet," I sputtered. "We haven't really . . ."

"Then get on the stick, son," Minnie replied firmly. "Use the media to maintain the moral high ground. Keep old what's his name constantly squirming."

"Benson."

"What?" Minnie said. It was obvious her mind was already three jumps ahead.

"Supervisor Benson," I replied. "Old what's his name. The one we want to squirm."

"The person doesn't matter," Minnie went on. "The principles are what's important. Keep the pressure on. Didn't you learn anything from Doctor King? What were you doing during the sixties, anyway?"

"I . . ."

"Listening to Beatles music no doubt," Minnie continued, shaking her head. "And probably weaving flowers in your hair. Well, things were different in the South. Now pay attention."

It was truly miraculous. For the next half hour Minnie Osbourne was reborn. As if by sheer force of will, her mind seemed to reintegrate itself as she regaled me with stories about the civil rights movement and the political battles waged by black Americans. She was precise, insightful, and erudite. I was astonished. I was also ashamed.

I was ashamed because I thought of all the time I'd spent with Minnie. All the time I hadn't taken her as seriously as I should have. Because she was old and forgetful I guess I assumed she'd always been that way. I'd let her diagnosis of Alzheimer's disease focus my attention on what she'd forgotten instead of what she still remembered. Minnie Osbourne wasn't a woman deserving of my pity. She was deserving of my respect.

My feelings aside, our voting drive now had some real steam. We had a leader. We had a chance. We had Minnie Osbourne.

III

Over the next few weeks, in addition to my regular ward duties I consulted daily with Minnie about our campaign. She was a seemingly endless stream of good ideas. Twice a week, voter registration tables were set up in our waiting area. We had a bake sale to raise money for envelopes, stamps, and lapel buttons. We bought placards and paint. A news conference was scheduled to kick things off.

During this time the entire hospital began to take on a whole new feeling. The place seemed to come to life. The staff smiled more. People shook hands. And the patients never looked better. During the day they happily lettered signs, stuffed mailers, and addressed labels. Each time I saw them line up for their medication, I began to have a twinge of uncomfortable doubt. I wasn't entirely certain what made people well any more.

It was during one of my afternoon strategy sessions with Minnie that I happened to see an attendant pass by in the hall with a new patient. I knew Dr. Lincoln was scheduled to accept admissions that day, so I had no idea why this young black woman struck me so. But she did. Perhaps it was her age, no more than eighteen at best, or that she seemed so tiny and frail, trembling as she was like a fragile flower. I stood and went to the door. The woman was escorted to a room a few doors away.

Then I spotted Alice Lincoln outside the nursing station. She had a chart in her hands. I excused myself from Minnie and walked toward Dr. Lincoln. Normally fairly stoic, Alice had a concerned look on her face.

"New patient?" I said, nodding.

"Real horror story," Dr. Lincoln said with a sigh as she closed the chart. "Her name is Neesha Graham. She's seventeen. Gang-raped in Griffith Park. The police found her naked and unconscious. I was on call last night and admitted her to the PES. When a bed opened up this morning I had her sent here. Her orders are already written, everything's done. Poor girl hasn't spoken a word to anyone. Sometimes I just don't . . ." Alice said as her voice trailed off. Then she turned and hurriedly wiped a tear from the corner of one eye. I knew she was really struggling.

We both stood silently for a moment. Then it hit me. "Would you mind if someone else took over the case?" I asked.

Alice looked puzzled. "I doubt if she'll open up to you," she said. "Besides, it's my turn to . . ."

"It wasn't me I had in mind," I replied. Then we were quiet again.

"I wouldn't mind at all," Dr. Lincoln finally said with a smile. "Not at all."

I rang Dr. Ashwin's home from the nursing station. I was taking a long shot and knew it. After three rings the phone was answered and not by a machine.

"Anita," I said. "This is Steve Seager. Would you do me a favor?"

IV

I stayed late at the hospital that night. Dr. Ashwin had been noncommittal over the phone. She said she just wasn't sure yet. I said we needed her. Then I waited. By eight o'clock I'd given up. I felt sad for everyone. And I was mad at myself as well. I had no right to pressure Anita Ashwin like that, I thought, after all she'd been through. No doubt, I was certain, I'd only made matters worse.

Collecting my lab coat and car keys, I closed the door to my small office, checked on Neesha Graham as I had done twice during the day, and slowly walked away. The hospital was quiet. My heels on the floor were the only sounds in the hallway. I knew it would be a long drive home.

Just as there had been that first morning when I arrived on the ward, as I got to the locked door a face was staring back at me through the little window. I quickly opened the door.

"I couldn't bring myself to turn the key," Dr. Ashwin said softly, sadly. "I just couldn't do it."

I touched her arm. "How long have you been standing out here?" I asked quietly.

Anita shook her head and gave me a faint smile. "Not long," she sighed, "but it feels like forever."

I waited for what I thought was the right moment. "Your patient is ready," I said finally.

Anita reached down and gave my hand a squeeze. Then she walked back onto Ward Three. "Thank you," she said.

I took the long way home that night. Going a few miles past my usual freeway exit, I ended up in Hermosa Beach, a small oceanside town just west of my South Bay home. Pulling my car to a stop next to the sand, I rolled down the window and took a few slow breaths. The air was marvelously wet and cool. A bright moon shone in one undisturbed circle far out on the smooth black water. Everything seemed so peaceful and calm. So unreal. I leaned back and closed my eyes. The Bin was a thousand miles away.

Then two sirens suddenly rang out in the distance. And everything came rushing back. With a start I sat up and collected myself. Shaking my head I turned the ignition, kicked the car in gear, and sped back to reality.

I don't know how long Anita talked to that poor young woman that night or if they even talked at all. But I know some healing went on. When I got back to Ward Three early the following morning, Dr. Ashwin was sleeping in a chair beside Neesha Graham's bed. And she was back at work every day from then on. Neesha Graham spoke to the nurses for the first time that day.

FIVE

LIES UNDER OATH

I

"I'M HEARING VOICES," the man said in a thick but understandable Hispanic accent.

It was very late. I was on call for the third night that week. It was mid-September, the end of summer. The air was hot and heavy. Our triage interview room seemed smaller than usual. "I see," I replied, mustering all of my dwindling supply of enthusiasm. "And what are these voices saying?"

The man seemed momentarily taken aback but quickly regained his composure. After pausing a second to collect his thoughts, he said, "The voices are telling me to kill myself."

I stared at him. He stared uncomfortably back at me. When I finally nodded my head, the man visibly relaxed. The rest of the interview went quickly. I admitted the man to the PES and arranged for him to go to Ward Three.

For a psychiatrist at The Bin this kind of story was standard stuff. I was fairly certain the man was lying. But with any person claiming to be suicidal, especially those who say voices are commanding them to complete the act, you have to be extra careful. Unfortunately, the street people know this, too. So, whenever someone, for whatever reason, wants into the hospital, they know how to get a ticket.

After only a few months of training, I'd begun to sense the difference between the true mentally ill and people only pretending to be insane. It's not a difference I can put into words. It's like trying to describe the taste of salt. You just have to try some.

Modern-day public psychiatry is faced with numerous moral and ethical issues unheard of in previous generations. One of the problems centers on this point: Most people who are mentally ill and desperately in need of institutional care don't want it. In fact, the majority will not even admit that they're sick. On the other hand, there is a growing number of people—the homeless, desperate, and hungry—who actively seek hospitalization. They will gladly endure blood tests, rigid regulations, and even medication if it means hot meals and a clean place to sleep.

The task of sorting through these people falls to psychiatrists at facilities like The Bin. We are the gatekeepers. We must decide who gets in and who stays out. As the year wore on, this was a decision that became increasingly more difficult and personally taxing to make.

If you are not mentally ill, so says the county, you do not belong in a mental hospital. It's a waste of good tax dollars. On the other hand, try escorting an old woman out the door who hasn't eaten for two days and is sleeping in a cemetery.

The man I admitted that night was Juan Cruz. As we sat in my office up on Ward Three the next morning, he laid his cards directly on the table. He apologized for saying he'd heard voices. It was something, he said, his brother-in-law had told him to do.

"I had nowhere else to turn," Juan said, his eyes never leaving mine. "You're my last hope."

I leaned forward a bit in my chair. "I'm not sure I understand," I said. "Last hope for what?"

"To ever see my wife and children again," Juan replied calmly. "You are my only chance to stay alive."

I spent a long time with Juan that session. I discovered we were almost the same age. That we enjoyed similar interests. To my amazement I learned that Juan was also a physician. Back home Dr. Cruz had been a prominent surgeon. We were alike in so many ways. Except the one that mattered. I had been born in the United States. Juan, on the other hand, was from El Salvador where he had, unfortunately, taken sides in a sensitive political dispute. There was now a price on his head.

Dr. Cruz had left El Salvador without official papers. He'd spent the last two years working as the night manager for a local 7-Eleven. One evening, he said, he'd been recognized. He came to The Bin the day he received deportation papers from the INS.

"If you release me I'm a dead man," Juan said, shaking his head.

As I mentioned, state law says I can keep a person fourteen days after his initial three-day detainment expires. Each fourteen-day hold is reviewed by the Superior Court who send officers called "referees" to the hospital where the proceedings are held—generally, in an empty conference room. Any further involuntary confinement must be done through a legal process called "conservatorship."

Conservatorship is a drastic process. Basically, the court is petitioned to declare a person incompetent to make decisions concerning his life. Another person, usually a relative—the "conservator"—is then appointed to make such decisions. Once declared incompetent, a person loses the right, without consent of the conservator, to enter into any type of contract, loan agreement, or mortgage. They cannot marry or start a divorce action, drive a car, handle their own money or property, or practice their profession. In short, they are declared a child again.

Juan asked that I file a conservatorship application for him. "But you'll never practice medicine again," I stuttered. By now my emotions were in a hopeless tangle.

Juan gave me a faint smile. Then he reached over and touched my arm. "My friend," he said quietly, "what would you do in my position?"

Of course, Juan Cruz did not belong in a mental hospital. But he didn't deserve to face a death squad, either. After his three days were up, I placed Juan on a fourteen-day hold. It would be four days before the Superior Court review hearing. I knew I would need the time to think this thing through. I also knew I needed some sound advice.

Every psychiatrist-in-training is assigned what is called a "supervisor." Your supervisor is a senior staff psychiatrist with whom you discuss the treatment of your patients. Your supervisor is also someone you can go to with personal matters. He is your official guide and mentor. My supervisor was Dr. Harold Jefferson, a well-respected, middle-aged psychoanalyst. I made an appointment to see Dr. Jefferson for the morning of Juan Cruz's review hearing.

II

In psychiatry, as in life, inspiration often comes from unexpected sources. And so it was with the case of Juan Cruz.

For the next few days I could think of little else but the upcoming hearing. "Your mind's off somewhere else today, son," Minnie Osbourne said midway through our daily political strategy/psychotherapy session.

"Sorry," I replied, snapping back to the task at hand.

"You having problems?" Minnie asked sincerely.

"I am, Minnie," I sighed. "I've got a decision to make. It involves an ethical choice and possibly someone's life."

"I see," Minnie said softly, leaning back and nodding her head. Then we were both quiet for a moment. "When I was a young girl back in Louisiana," Minnie finally said, "my friend Ruthie Justice and I stole some candy from the general store. We were poor and that candy just looked so good. Anyway," she went on quietly, "the owner, a Mr. Ferguson—the biggest white man I'd ever seen then or since—caught me walking home with part of that candy still in my pocket. He knew I'd been with another girl and demanded to know who she was. He lectured me about stealing and the importance of always telling the truth. He said if I didn't give him my friend's name he would tell my daddy and see to it that I got a whipping I'd never forget."

Minnie's face turned distant. A small tear welled in the corner of one eye. "I was terrified," she went on. "I was scared for myself and the beating I might get. So I told him Ruthie's name."

Minnie took in a breath to clear her mind. "Of course," she said, now much more in control, "Mr. Ferguson told both our parents, anyway. Ruthie's father was a drinking man. He beat her so hard he broke her leg." Minnie sighed again. "To this day I'm still ashamed of what I did," she said finally.

Then Minnie reached over and gently took my hand. "Go with your heart, son," she said quietly. "Let the good Lord sort out the right and wrong of it. You'll sleep better, I promise you."

After sitting and holding Minnie's hand for what seemed like a silent eternity, I did something I'd never done with a patient before. I leaned over and kissed her on the cheek.

I canceled my appointment with Dr. Jefferson. Juan Cruz's review hearing came and went. Juan told the court referee that he was hearing voices and I said I believed him. The referee upheld the hospital's hold. "Thank you," Juan said quietly as we walked back to the ward. I only nodded.

I knew I'd done the right thing but still I couldn't ignore a growing knot in the pit of my stomach. Lying to a hearing referee in a hospital conference room was one thing, I knew, but lying in front of a Superior Court judge in a state court house was definitely another. And I knew that situation awaited me. I filed conservatorship papers on Juan Cruz the morning after his hearing. A court date was set. A court date that would include the INS. That would include attorneys. That would include that judge. It was a court date on which I would have to step forward and face my own Mr. Ferguson.

III

It took quite a jolt to get my mind off the problems with Juan Cruz and back to the affairs of Ward Three. As usual, for The Bin, of course, the next crisis was not far distant. The same day I filed Dr. Cruz's conservatorship papers I got a call from Martin Braga's mother. She was frantic. She said Martin had just phoned to tell her he was signing himself out of the hospital.

I found Martin in his room. He was collecting his things into a small satchel, the kind boys use to carry baseballs and gloves. He looked up briefly when I came in, then returned to his packing. I was confused. I couldn't get a feel for Martin's mood. I only knew something was terribly wrong.

"Are you going somewhere?" I asked, sitting on the edge of a small night table beside Martin's bed.

"Yeah," Martin said dryly. "I thought I'd take two weeks on the Riviera. The family does it every summer."

I was stunned by Martin's seemingly abrupt change. Over the months I thought he and I had truly formed a good relationship. I believed he was making real progress. He'd given every indication of having gained a deepening insight into himself. I thought he was

64

finally coming to grips with his disease. Now, in an instant, all that appeared to have changed. Just looking at his face and listening to the tone of his voice, I realized I didn't know Martin Braga at all.

"But what about your mother . . . ?" I sputtered.

"Fuck my mother!" Martin shouted, spinning on his heels to face me. "Fuck the hospital. Fuck therapy. Fuck this fucking disease. And fuck you, Doctor," he spat.

I was frozen. For a moment I thought Martin was going to attack me. He must have sensed my panic because after a few seconds of tense glaring his shoulders slowly dropped. "I'm sorry, Doctor Seager," he sighed. "I didn't mean that. You and the staff here have been very kind to me. It's just time I left, that's all. It's time to get on with my life, whatever that is."

"But you've come such a long way," I said finally. "And I—I mean *we* have more work to do yet. There are still things to . . ." I said, then stopped short. Martin had a small smile on his face. Shaking my head I smiled back.

Whatever else can be said about schizophrenics, they can, at times, be incredibly perceptive. Martin had instantly caught my slip. I was both embarrassed and strangely enlightened at the same time. Looking at Martin's smile I suddenly realized why I wanted him to stay. It wasn't for his benefit. It was for mine.

I wanted Martin Braga to get as well as he possibly could because it made me feel good. The more he improved, the more competent I felt. I wanted to continue basking in the glory of a job well done. Martin wanted to get out and live his life.

"Where will you go?" I asked finally.

Martin went back to his packing. His smile was gone. He had that robot look in his eyes again. "Home for a while. Then maybe back to school," he said flatly.

"Will you take your medication?" I asked. This was a key issue. For schizophrenics with insight into their disease, medication takes on a symbolic meaning quite apart from any therapeutic gains it might provide. It is a continual reminder that they're ill. That they're no longer in control. It reminds them of a great many things, I suppose.

When Martin hesitated for a moment I knew we were in for trouble. "Of course I'll take it," he replied flatly. "I'm mentally ill. I need it, don't I?"

Martin and I spoke for a few more minutes, but I can't recall what was said. I do remember, however, how much my heart ached as I watched him finish packing that little bag. I remember how deeply impressed I was with the real tragedy of mental illness. At that moment, I realized that despite my most heartfelt desire, medication, and support, Martin Braga was not going to get much better than he was right at that moment. And that in all probability he would gradually get worse. That one day it might be him, my friend, at the dumpster behind the supermarket. Sadly, I think this was something Martin had come to realize some time ago.

"Thanks, Doc," Martin said after I'd gotten his discharge papers done and phoned his mother to explain the situation. We were standing just outside the door to Ward Three.

"They'll see you in outpatient clinic in a month," I said as we shook hands and Martin turned to go.

I felt completely empty as I watched Martin Braga walk slowly down the hallway. I knew I would never see him again.

IV

I was feeling depressed and suddenly very tired after saying goodbye to Martin Braga. He was the first patient who'd given me a real look into mental illness. He'd made me see things from his point of view. He'd shared some of his suffering. He had touched me.

I walked back into my office, locked the door, and collapsed into the chair behind my desk. Slumping down I closed my eyes and let my mind drift. Every bone in my body ached.

Sinking lower in the chair, I slowly began to retrace the beginning three months of my internship. Images of patients' faces and bits of conversation appeared and then eerily floated away. Soon everything was just a hazy blur. Then I remembered my first night on call. And I remembered Mr. Thompson, Harry Houdini. Instantly I was sitting straight and wide awake. "Jesus," I said to myself. "What in hell ever happened to that guy?"

While initially there had been so much apprehension and mystery concerning his disappearance, as time went on there was less and less talk about him. We never received a call from concerned relatives. We never heard a word from anybody. Finally, I guess, everyone just forgot the man. I know I had. "Jesus," I mumbled out loud again.

The monthly staff meeting was held in a conference room just outside the PES. It was a session in which faculty, staff, and residents met to air grievances, formulate policy, and generally confer. The meeting was chaired by the Boss, our department's chief of psychiatry, Dr. Noel Maxwell, and, as such, was very dignified and formal. Dr. Maxwell, a distinguished black man of fifty-five, was a nationally respected psychiatrist and author of one of the better texts on treatment of mental illness. I and the other residents were in awe of him. We felt it an honor simply to be invited to his monthly sessions.

It happened soon after the meeting was called to order. Dr. Maxwell, dressed in his signature dark silk suit and striped tie, was presenting a proposal for a major overhaul of the PES physical structure. "I think with a different layout we can work more efficiently," he said to the respectfully hushed audience.

"I disagree," a voice said. We all stared at one another. We stared at Dr. Maxwell who stared right back at us.

Then everyone in the room jumped when, suddenly, with a loud crack, a foot appeared through the ceiling followed by a shower of latheboard and plaster. In a crash, Mr. Thompson, our long-lost patient, dropped like a stone into the center of the conference room table.

"Things around here are just fine," he continued without missing a beat. "This joint is much better than the last dump I was in. Besides, the FBI's radar can't reach me here."

It took a moment for the dust to settle and for Mr. Thompson to get himself straightened up. Everyone's eyes were wide as dinner plates. There wasn't a closed mouth in the room. Except for Dr. Maxwell, that is.

"Thank you for your input, sir," he said smoothly with just the barest hint of a smile. "What do the rest of you think?" he added.

SIX

THE DEAD RISE

I

AFTER HOSPITAL SECURITY had Mr. Thompson firmly in tow, the normally staid staff meeting erupted into mild pandemonium. We laughed until we cried. Even Dr. Maxwell got caught up in it. As soon as things threatened to die down, someone would point to the huge hole in the ceiling and the whoops would start all over again. Finally, after five full minutes everyone was sighing, smiling, and wiping their faces. At The Bin, a good laugh was hard to come by. For a few warm moments we all felt close.

At last, running a white handkerchief over his face, Dr. Maxwell stood. "Hell, let's all go home," he said and the room broke out in one final, united cheer.

It took the maintenance people two days of creeping through the hospital's elaborate airduct system to map out all of Mr. Thompson's three-month stay in the ceiling. And another day at least to catalogue all the items he'd taken back up with him from his nightly forays into the hospital proper.

After somehow shedding his restraints, it seems Mr. Thompson had initially pushed up a small section of the checkerboard-style ceiling panels that first night in the PES and had just pulled himself on up. Once he'd mastered the technique, he basically came and went as he pleased.

"The main duct is furnished better than my house," one of the men said as, incredibly, he lowered the second of three office chairs to the ground. I was on call that night and had been watching the men work for a while. I could only stare in disbelief at those chairs. My feelings turned to amazement and admiration when the final items—a mattress, box springs and bed frame—were slowly handed down.

While the staff was delighted to retrieve their lost objects that had so mysteriously disappeared over the months, everyone was left with the same question: How had Mr. Thompson done it? A full bed frame? The entire week he was with us before going to the state hospital, we asked him every day. And never once did we get an answer.

II

As what passed for autumn descended on southern California and October rolled around, things were changing on Ward Three. Carl Williams, my alien from Zano, got about as good as we figured he was going to get. He'd managed to stay reasonably well groomed for a few weeks. He was taking his medication without protest and, aside from an occasional reference to "Kirk and the men," was behaving fairly rationally, so arrangements were made for his placement in a nearby board-and-care home. As he left, I shook his hand and wished him well. "Take your medicine," I said as he shuffled happily away.

"You bet," Carl said, turning for a moment. Then he winked at me.

"See you back in for Christmas," I sighed under my breath as I closed and locked the ward door.

As always at The Bin, no sooner had one patient vacated his bed than it was filled again by another. An hour after Carl's winking goodbye, we were notified that someone was on his way up. When any new patient arrived on the ward, there was always some disruption, a slightly altered routine. But this time it would be different. This time things would take a very bizarre turn. A turn that none of us could ever have imagined was coming.

When a patient was discharged, his bed got stripped and the floors thoroughly mopped. The nurses saw to the bed. The floors were done by the janitor. Our janitor was Ben Smith. Our janitor had always, it seemed, been Ben Smith.

Ben was working on Ward Three when I arrived at The Bin in July. But so, apparently, had he been when everyone else I knew arrived as well. I asked Nurse Fisher just before she retired from twenty years of county service if she remembered when Ben had first begun work at the hospital. "He's been here as long as me," Mrs. Fisher replied, shaking her head. "And Hattie Rivers says he was here with her, too. Hattie Rivers worked ten years before my time."

Ben Smith was a true black southern gentleman. He was unfailingly courteous—always with a kind word for everyone, patient or staff—religiously prompt, and had never, as best anyone could recall, missed a day of work. You could set your watch by the man. Ben Smith was as much a part of Ward Three as the walls and furniture.

That's why the arrival of our new patient caused such a stir. Oliver Carson was a thin black man in his seventies. Mr. Carson arrived in a wheelchair pushed by an orderly. Mr. Carson, I read from his chart, had suddenly become combative at a rest home, trying to run his chair through a plate glass window, then setting fire to another man's bed sheets. This, of course, guaranteed an admission ticket to The Bin.

Ben Smith had just finished mopping Carl Williams's old room when Mr. Carson was wheeled by the door. I was standing in the hallway. Suddenly I heard a mop handle clatter to the floor. Thinking perhaps Ben had fallen, I quickly ran down the corridor.

Ben was standing against the far wall next to a window. His mop was at his feet. He was frozen. He looked terrified.

"Are you alright, Ben?" I said, slowly walking over. Ben didn't reply. Only when I touched his arm did he startle back to reality.

"Excuse me, Doctor Seager," he mumbled, "I've got to go." Then, leaving his mop and bucket behind, he ran from the room. He looked like a man who'd seen a ghost.

After a stunned moment I followed behind Ben as quickly as I could. I heard the ward door slam shut. When I finally made it there myself and looked into the outside hallway, Ben was nowhere in sight.

No one saw or heard from Ben the rest of the day. He missed work the next morning. And the next. By the third day we all became truly concerned.

After rounds on Friday Ben was the only thing on everyone's mind.

"Shouldn't we call his family?" Miss Givens asked.

"I've never heard Ben mention a family," Dr. Ashwin said. "Has anyone?"

There were seven of us in the room. No one had a reply.

"There must be someone to call," Dr. Lamb, the psychologist, added. "He must have a home. He has to go somewhere at night."

"I'll check with personnel," I said finally. "I'll tell them it's an emergency. They'll have an address or phone number."

"Let us know," Miss Givens said quietly. "I'm worried about that old man."

It was a couple of hours before I had the time to slip away to my office and phone downstairs. My call was answered on the third ring.

"Personnel," a young woman's bright voice said.

I explained our problem and asked if she wouldn't check her files for a way to contact Ben. She put me on hold. After two anxious minutes she returned. I had pen and paper in hand.

"The name was Benjamin Smith?" the woman asked.

"Correct."

"And you say he works in the maintenance department?"

I didn't like the feeling I was getting. "He's worked here at least thirty years," I said warily.

"I'm sorry," the young woman replied. "I've got no record of a Benjamin Smith in maintenance or any other department."

"There must be some mistake," I stuttered.

"I'm sorry, sir," the woman persisted. "There's no record of any Benjamin Smith ever working for the county."

"Thank you," I said, then slowly put the phone down.

III

When I told the staff that afternoon, their response was the same as mine had been. When I assured them there was no mistake, we all just quietly stared at one another.

"That old fool better be here on Monday," Miss Givens said finally. "So I can chew out his lazy butt." She was just as scared as the rest of us.

There was a strange sense of foreboding that next Monday morning as the clock crept toward nine and we still had no Ben Smith. Rounds began ten minutes later. Everyone, including Dr. Singh, was unusually quiet. No one knew quite what to say or how to feel. We were all frightened and confused.

But it didn't last long, for me, anyway. At nine-thirty I got called out of the room. Someone wanted me on the phone. I didn't think of Ben Smith for a few days after that.

I took the call in the nursing station. The Superior Court was on the line. They'd moved Juan Cruz's conservatorship hearing up to Wednesday, the day after tomorrow.

It was all getting to be too much. I returned to rounds but nothing sunk in. I couldn't get the ominous specter of that courtroom and a black-robed judge out of my mind. When the group broke up I was first out the door. "I'll be back," I shouted over my shoulder to no one in particular.

I needed some time to think, to sort things out. So I went where I always went when life at The Bin heated up. It was a secret place Dr. Ashwin had shown me. I could use it, she said, only if I swore myself to secrecy.

It was a little gem of emerald green, a small, hidden island of quiet beauty tucked away from the bleak, vicious ghetto. It was out behind the maintenance building, a structure that had once been part of the main hospital, serving as a huge psychiatric ward. It was surrounded by a tall fence.

Inside was a tended lawn that sloped gently in the middle. Thick-limbed trees had been carefully planted to give the illusion of a country walking lane. There were flowers. There were wooden benches for quiet conversation. If you listened carefully, you could hear the gentle call of an occasional small bird that had somehow escaped attack from the flock of enormous black crows that infested the network of powerlines near the hospital parking lot.

This idyllic piece of incongruent fairyland, Dr. Ashwin explained, had been built for patients of the old hospital ward. Back, apparently, she added, when a few people actually cared about mentally ill human beings. It had continued to be tended, I surmised, because it was probably on a county crew's work list and had simply never been removed.

After my phone call from the court that morning, I retreated to my secret spot. To think. To sort. To wonder.

I went back to work sometime that afternoon. I know I was there the next day, too, because a week later I saw that I'd written notes on all my charts. But I don't recall anything of the days. I was on automatic pilot. My mind was consumed with Juan Cruz.

I considered discussing my problem with my supervisor. I thought of Dr. Ashwin as well. And finally my wife. But in the end I decided against any of them. Strangely, after all was said and done, I knew that were I ever to be at peace with myself, really at peace, I had to face this one alone.

I stopped by to see Juan Cruz late Tuesday night before going home and explained everything to him again. All the while I was seeing that judge and rehearsing the lies inside my head. "Are you certain you know what you're doing?" I asked, standing to leave.

Dr. Cruz gave me a knowing, compassionate smile. His voice was tinged with emotion. "Are *you* sure you know what *you're* doing?" he said quietly.

I saw Juan Cruz briefly the next morning in the crowded corridor of the cavernous downtown Superior Court building. He was dressed in green hospital-issue scrubs. An attendant stood with him. Neither of us spoke as we passed. Taking a deep breath I pushed open the huge wooden doors and walked into the courtroom.

Unfortunately, it was all just as I'd imagined and dreaded it would be. My heart beat like a trip-hammer the whole time. When the judge was announced, I couldn't look up. The cases previous to ours seemed to take hours. Then the bailiff called "Juan Cruz" and I was asked to take the stand.

In all the days of self-imposed torture I'd endured over this issue, when I think of it today the one image I still come back to is the picture of Minnie Osbourne's forthright, noble face as she told the story about Mr. Ferguson. And I always hear her words, "Go with your heart." That image and those words were with me as I sat in the witness box and raised my right hand.

And, of course, Minnie was right. Once I'd gotten my heart

straight, the whole matter went quite easily. I said Juan Cruz was hearing voices and he agreed with me. I said he was a continual danger to himself and Juan agreed again. I said he was clearly incapable of caring for himself and again Juan concurred. Juan's court-appointed attorney asked a few perfunctory questions and it was over. Juan wept when his conservatorship was granted. Then they recessed for lunch.

It hurts me to think of Juan Cruz, such an intelligent, educated, and capable man, stuck in some state hospital spending his days making leather belts or gluing pictures. But then I consider the alternative. In my heart I know I did right.

IV

Of course my sense of relief was tremendous once the Juan Cruz affair had finally come to an end. But this was short-lived. The other dilemma faced me first thing back at work on Thursday. There was still no sign of Ben Smith. I knew something had to give, and soon, so I acted on a hunch. It was something I should have done days ago. Although Mr. Carson, our new man in the wheelchair, was Dr. Ashwin's patient, I asked if I might interview him alone. I was the only one who'd seen Ben Smith's strange reaction to his arrival. I had no idea what the connection was. But I knew there was one. When I found out, it was my turn to be stunned. My turn to run from the room and down the hall.

Oliver Carson, bent and thinned with age, had a few tufts of gray, scouring-pad hair around his ears and an enormous, warm smile. Mr. Carson suffered from bipolar disorder. He'd stopped taking his lithium, which led to the board-and-care incident, then to The Bin. And finally to my small office where he and I chatted that morning.

Oliver Carson, Miss Givens told me, had been in and out of our hospital for as long as anyone could remember. "He's probably been a patient here longer than Ben Smith's been janitor," she added.

A half hour later as I watched an orderly return Mr. Carson to his room, I tried to convince myself that his story made sense. But I didn't have much time for thinking. I was quickly out the ward door and down the hall.

I rode the elevator to the basement where the hospital kept its records. Records of all the people who'd ever worked at County General. And records of all its patients as well.

SEVEN

THE SWORD OF GOD

I

"BEN?" I called out into the darkness. "Ben?" I said again but got no reply. Beside me in the dark basement boiler room, Dr. Ashwin shone a flashlight under heavy metal pipes and into dank, dust-filled corners. I'd confided Ben's secret to Anita. After Juan Cruz I'd had enough of carrying burdens alone.

It seemed like we'd been stumbling through the dingy, tomb-like hospital basement for hours. We'd clamored over old rusted machines, crawled under wet ledges, and jumped at the sight of a skittering rat. It was nearly midnight and we were both very tired of breathing musty air and listening to the distant sound of eerie, moaning metal.

Then Dr. Ashwin saw it. And we both heard a small scuffling noise. Swinging the flashlight beam alongside a huge, empty cauldron, there was the tip of a frayed hospital blanket. We glanced at one another, then carefully headed over.

"Hello, Ben," I said with a combination of relief and astonishment. Behind that antiquated boiler, hidden from decades of view, was Ben Smith's home. Inside an alcove sunk into the wall was a bed, a nightstand, and a clothes rack on which were hung two neatly pressed maintenance uniforms. Most amazingly, however, were the books. There were stacks of them. They filled almost every square inch of empty floor, save a small pathway leading away from the bed.

And on that bed was Ben Smith. "May we come in?" I asked as Ben shifted his legs and sat. Then he clicked on a small night-table lamp. Anita touched a stack of books. "Have you read all these?" she asked quietly.

"They passed a lot of lonely hours," Ben replied. Then we were all silent again.

"You haven't been outside this hospital in thirty years, have you, Ben?" I asked.

Ben sighed and stared at the floor for a moment. Then he looked back up at me. "No, sir, I haven't," he said quietly. "I surely haven't."

II

Ben almost seemed relieved to finally tell his story, to finally share it all with someone. "I had my first breakdown at twenty-eight," he began slowly. Then he smiled. "I wasn't always an old man, you know," he continued. "When I was younger I could cut it up with the ladies pretty good. Even have me a son out there somewhere." We both smiled back. Then Ben's face sagged again. "Yeah, I was pretty good until the voices started," he said sadly.

"That was before you doctors had all those medicines," Ben went on. "So when you came to a place like this, you just stayed." Ben's voice drifted off. He was staring over my shoulder. "Things were pretty bad back then," he said quietly.

Suddenly my heart ached. I'd read *The Snake Pit*.

"But how did you ever become a janitor?" Dr. Ashwin asked.

"I've always been a janitor," Ben stated. "Right from the start."

"I don't understand," I said.

"Back then all the patients had jobs," Ben replied. "It kept us busy and saved the state a fair bit of money."

"Some things never change," I added, and Ben grinned again.

"Then the attorneys and judges got involved with mental health and people started being sent out of here," Ben went on. "I got real scared." Again Ben was quiet for a moment. "I saw how those boys lived out there," he sighed. "They'd come back so filthy and raggedy. Or I'd read where one got stabbed or starved to death. Well, you know," Ben nodded. "Like they do now." We both nodded back.

"Anyway, I didn't want any part of that," Ben continued. "So I kept on being a janitor. And one day I just took up living down here."

"Who else knew you were down here?" I asked in amazement.

"Some of the other patients knew, but I guess they never said anything," Ben said, his voice trailing off a bit. "I'd hoped by now they'd have all died or drifted away. But I guess not." Ben's eyes suddenly turned hard. "Ollie Carson told you to look for me down here, didn't he?" he asked, and I nodded. "That man never could keep quiet about anything," Ben said, shaking his head.

"And nobody from the hospital caught on to you all these years?" Dr. Ashwin asked.

Ben shook his head. "Not until today," he sighed sadly. Then he stood and started gathering his things together.

"What are you doing?" Anita asked.

"I guess I'll have to be leaving now," Ben said, neatly folding his uniforms into a pile. "I hear some of those board-and-care homes aren't so bad."

Again, Dr. Ashwin and I looked at one another. "I think they're down a patient on Ward One," she said. "We could transfer Mr. Carson there."

"And we need a good janitor on Ward Three," I said. "Someone who already knows the place."

"I don't understand," Ben said, stopping his folding and turning to face us.

"Ben," Anita said, taking the old man's hands. "I don't know what's right or wrong here. But I do know," she continued, "a man shouldn't be forced out of the only home he's known for thirty years. We need you on Ward Three. Come back," she said, squeezing Ben's hands. "Nothing will be said to anyone. I promise."

Ben looked at me and I nodded. Then he tried to speak but stopped. He tried a second time but stopped again. Finally, after taking a minute to compose himself, he stood up straight. "I thank you both very kindly," he said in a voice just barely under control. "But now I'll have to ask you to leave, please. It's not proper for a grown man to cry in front of a lady."

Ben returned to work the next morning. There were a few questions, which he deflected with a smile. Mr. Carson was sent to Ward One, and after a few days the entire incident was forgotten. And for the rest of my time on Ward Three we had the cleanest floors of anyone, anywhere.

III

November was coming up and this meant two things. Thanksgiving was in the offing. But that was the least significant of the two. November also meant election day and the culmination of our hard-fought voter registration drive.

Given what we had to work with and who we were trying to mobilize, I thought we'd done marvelously well. According to my sources, with only two weeks to go, we had nearly five thousand new voters on the district's roles. I was elated. Minnie Osbourne, the master strategist, however, wasn't so sure.

"Registering is one thing," she said as she settled into the chair across the desk from me in my office. "Actually getting people to vote is quite another."

This was an angle I hadn't considered. "What do you mean?" I asked. "Why would they register and then not vote?"

Minnie laughed and patted my hand. "You poor boy," she said sweetly. "All those years in school. Missed the class in common sense, did you?"

I laughed, too. I truly loved that old woman. "I guess I did," I replied chuckling.

"Registering is the easy part," Minnie went on, now quite serious again. "Do you have busses arranged to take these people to the polls?"

I was getting a sinking feeling. "There really isn't money and I didn't . . ." I said, but was cut off.

"Will your people be there to explain the ballot?"

"I hadn't . . ."

"Can they operate the lever machines?"

"I don't . . ."

"Will they be allowed in the polling places?" Minnie continued, her voice rising. "Is there a poll tax? Will they claim the registration lists are lost?" It was obvious Minnie wasn't paying attention to me any more. Her dim eyes were burning. She wasn't in my office. She was back in Louisiana. Back to a time when these issues were much bigger than Supervisor Benson or freeways.

And then Minnie started coughing. The spell didn't last long but it wracked her tiny body. I was scared.

"Are you alright?" I asked, leaning over to touch Minnie's shoulder.

"I'm fine," she said, nodding her head and smiling.

"How long have you had that cough?" I asked.

"It's nothing," she said firmly. "Now where were we?"

I waited a moment before speaking. "You were asking about rides to the voting booths and poll taxes and lost registration lists," I said hesitantly. I didn't like the look in Minnie's eyes.

"Don't be silly," she said brightly. "We fought those battles years ago. Where did a young man like you hear about poll taxes anyway?"

The voter registration drive was now the last thing on my mind. After escorting Minnie back to her room, I called a friend from the medicine department and asked if he could stop over and see her.

When I mentioned this to Miss Givens, she didn't look surprised. "Reports from the night shift say Minnie's started to wander," she said. "They found her cleaning the dayroom at three this morning. Thought she was back in New Orleans. Said she had to finish before the lady of the house got back."

We both stared down the hall toward Minnie's room. "Oh, Jesus," I sighed.

IV

I mentioned that at County General a good laugh was hard to come by. Basically, mental illness just isn't funny. But there are those rare moments.

Ironically, the patient who replaced Mr. Carson after his transfer to Ward One was also in a wheelchair. Edwin Lightwater, however, was a much younger man and, except for the chair, appeared to be in pretty good health.

Mr. Lightwater said he'd hurt his back a few years ago in an industrial accident, the exact details of which were a bit vague. Mr. Lightwater also lived in a board-and-care home. At sporadic intervals he would wheel himself out the door and take to the road. He'd always get picked up miles from home. Occasionally, however, he refused to tell the police where he lived. And this meant only one thing: The Bin.

I'm not much of a practical joker, but every so often it's the only thing that'll do. To understand the joke, however, you have to understand it's target. Florence Wilson was the nurse on Ward Three who took over for the evening after Miss Givens went home at three.

Mrs. Wilson was a large black woman in her mid-forties. When I first came to Ward Three, I knew her as a personable, pleasant, if somewhat benign woman. This all changed, however, during the fall. That autumn Florence Wilson got religion.

It was, she said, a real Saul-on-the-road-to-Damascus kind of thing. "Like I'd been hit in the head with a two-by-four," she added graphically. She'd been watching an evangelical television program, not really paying much attention, when the minister said something that caught her ear. By the end of that half hour she was a goner. The spiritual two-by-four had struck. "I'll never be the same," she said. And she was right.

While the staff was initially pleased to hear of Mrs. Wilson's conversion—much the same way you're pleased when anything perceived as good happens to someone you know—our opinion rapidly changed. Peaceful Nurse Wilson quickly became Florence Wilson, Sword of God.

She kept the nursing-area radio continually tuned to religious stations and not the quiet musical kind. She went in for the real hellfire stuff. She talked, nonstop, it seemed, about all the good God had done in her life and how much he could do for the "heathen hordes." When she started leaving pamphlets around the ward and kneeling to pray with patients at their bedside, we'd all had about enough.

Everyone tried talking some sense into her. We even had her supervisor come up. All to no avail. Rumor had it that her job was on the line. I liked Mrs. Wilson. She had children to support. Drastic measures were clearly called for.

Everything came together quite inadvertently. It involved me accidently seeing Mr. Lightwater one evening long after he supposed all the doctors had gone home. When I passed his door, he was standing in the middle of the floor. His radio was on. I think he was dancing. His wheelchair had been pushed into a corner.

I looked at Mr. Lightwater and Mr. Lightwater looked at me. We both immediately sensed the import of the moment. Acutely aware of the financial disaster that loomed with any sudden change in his disability status, Mr. Lightwater began to totter like a drunk, then made a comically spastic beeline for his chair.

Mr. Lightwater and I had a little talk that evening. In exchange for my silence, he promised me a favor.

The next afternoon, promptly at three, Mrs. Wilson and the rest of the evening staff were all in the nursing station just finishing reports, when I walked in and began thumbing through a chart. Mr. Lightwater was aimlessly wheeling himself around the corridor in front of the windows.

"You know, Mrs. Wilson," I began innocuously, "I'll admit at first I didn't pay much attention to all this religious stuff you've been talking about, but lately I think I'm beginning to have a change of heart."

Mrs. Wilson immediately perked up. The rest of the staff looked at me with combined curiosity and dread.

"Do you mean that, Doctor Seager?" Mrs. Wilson said hopefully.

"I certainly do," I replied. "I've finally gotten the Spirit."

"Praise God," Mrs. Wilson said, glancing skyward.

"Lord, not another one," someone whispered behind me.

"In fact," I said, laying the chart on the counter, "I don't think I can control myself any longer." As I walked toward the door, the astonished staff parted before me like the Red Sea.

I went out into the hallway. "Stop!" I shouted to Mr. Lightwater who'd just passed by. I stole a glance at the faces watching me through the window. There wasn't a closed mouth among them.

"Mr. Lightwater," I said solemnly, my right arm raised in the air. "Stand up and walk."

Mr. Lightwater was terrific. He played his part to the hilt. After feigning confusion, he made me repeat my request. "Stand up and walk," I said again with appropriate dignity and flair. Slowly and dramatically Mr. Lightwater rose from his wheelchair and after a few shaky steps confidently strode past me, walking down the hall and into his room.

In unison everyone in the nursing station let out a scream. Mrs. Wilson momentarily swooned. When I took a bow in their direction, however, the laughter started and wouldn't stop. Mrs. Wilson quickly came to her senses and, somewhat grudgingly at first, finally joined in as well.

Later that evening Mrs. Wilson and I had a long conversation. Of course, I apologized for my little stunt but then went on to explain the reasoning behind it. And for the first time in weeks she listened. For the first time in weeks that glaze was gone from her eyes. We parted as good friends.

To everyone's relief, our radio was soon back on soft rock. The theological lectures stopped and the pamphlets disappeared. We had our old Mrs. Wilson back.

V

Mark Riddel, my friend from medicine, was by to see Minnie Osbourne that same afternoon I called. All the while he was examining her, I was nervous as a cat.

"I think she has a touch of heart failure," Dr. Riddel said as we sat inside my office. "I started her on a diuretic. She should do fine," he added.

I was so relieved I could have cried. Dr. Riddel couldn't help but notice. "This lady special to you?" he asked.

"Very much so," I replied.

"She likes you, too," Dr. Riddel said with a smile. "She told me twice."

I said I was so relieved I could have cried. And after Dr. Riddel left my office, that's exactly what I did.

EIGHT

FRIENDS AND FAMILY

I

I SHOULD HAVE seen it coming but, of course, I didn't. I was just too close and cared too much. I was so clouded by how I wanted things to be that I never saw how they really were. This was, I learned, an occupational hazard of psychiatry. When you really know your patients well, you just naturally become attached. And this can sometimes color your view of them. It also makes the pain worse.

Other medical specialties operate on just the opposite principle. The system is designed to minimize closeness. Rounds are conducted at lightning speed. Doctors talk about patients rather than to them. Everything, it seems, is done by someone else with an expensive machine in another building. Bills are computerized. Charts audited. Discharge decisions made by insurance company formulas.

It's sort of a medical big bang theory. Doctors and patients, like bodies in the universe, are separating from one another at an ever-increasing velocity. This distancing, I know, is distressing to patients. We have, it seems, flung them like so many bobbing dinghys into an alien technological sea. Doctors, however, work from a different mode. It's not that they don't want to be close with patients; most, I'm sure, do. It just hurts so bad when something goes wrong as it inevitably does. Distance is safe and comforting. It must be something akin to being a bomber pilot. You know there are real people down there. It's just that they're so *far* down there.

II

With election day only a week away, I began to get truly excited. I was enormously proud of the way so many disparate people had pulled together toward a common goal. I was amazed at the dormant energy we'd harnassed. And, of course, I was pleased with our results. Busses or no busses, five thousand new voters was nothing to sneeze at.

And the closer we got to that first Tuesday in November, the stronger were the signals from Benson's people. The chinks in their armor had begun to show. I think they were nervous.

Supervisor Benson began to make daily appearances in the ghetto, something he'd previously done only episodically. But suddenly the man was everywhere, kissing babies, opening convenience stores, waving from open-topped cars. We started to wonder if he didn't have a twin.

Of course, Benson's escapades were the main topic of my daily sessions with Minnie. I wouldn't realize until later, however, that more and more, I was doing most of the talking.

"Benson's really running scared," I said two days before the election. Minnie only nodded.

"Do you believe he had the nerve to show his face at a mental health center?" I said with a sarcastic smile. "You can bet that picture will be plastered all over the front page tomorrow."

"It surely will," Minnie replied quietly.

I leaned back in my chair, running my hands through my hair. "Do you think we've done enough?" I sighed. "Do you think all this work will amount to anything?"

Minnie looked as if she were thinking. "Did my son call today?" she said finally. Her son, the lawyer, of course, had never phoned once.

I was taken aback for a moment. "No, Minnie, not today," I said.

"I see," she replied softly. "He's an attorney, you know."

I touched Minnie's hand across the desk. She suddenly looked so small and old. "Why don't we stop for today," I said. "I can see you're tired. Besides, I have one more meeting with the voting people and I'm already late."

I took Minnie back to her room, went to my meeting, saw the rest of my patients that afternoon, then drove the long way home. I wanted time to mull over the upcoming big event. I wracked my brain the entire way, trying to think of some stone we'd left unturned, some small detail yet to be sewn up.

I expected to see Big Daddy Benson's picture in the paper the next morning and I did. It was the headline, however, that shocked me: "Benson rescinds freeway plan" it read in bold letters. "Proposes increase in mental health budget," the smaller type said.

"We won!" I shouted, standing straight up at the breakfast table. My kids looked up from their cereal, glanced knowingly at each other, then returned to eating.

I was elated. Racing into the bedroom, I fumbled for my keys, grabbed my jacket, and flew toward the door. My wife, newspaper in hand, was waiting for me.

"Congratulations," she said and gave me a hug. "You've done a wonderful thing."

"Thank you," I said, "but it wasn't me."

There was one person who truly deserved thanks and I wanted to be the one to tell her. All the way to the hospital I tried to imagine the look on Minnie Osbourne's face when I read her the paper.

It was just past eight as I pulled into the hospital parking lot, scaring up a small band of crows perched on the tire stop in my parking space. I grabbed my paper, jumped out of the car, and jogged across the pavement.

"Good job," the sign-in clerk said as I hustled by toward an open elevator car. "Thank you," I shouted back as the doors closed.

The ride to the third floor seemed to take forever. County General was notorious for its creaky equipment and our elevator system was exhibit A. I imagined a little man downstairs straining with a pulley.

At last the doors opened again and I trotted down the hall to Ward Three. I was so excited I dropped my keys. Once inside I relocked the door and made a beeline for the nursing station. I was disappointed to find it empty.

Pausing a moment to catch my breath, I walked down to Minnie Osbourne's room. I was grinning from ear to ear.

I saw it just before I got to the door. I can't exactly describe what I felt but I knew I couldn't move another step. I'd suddenly been turned to granite. I was staring into the corner of Minnie Osbourne's room. The corner where Ben Smith's mop bucket sat.

Somehow I finally summoned the courage to move into the doorway. The newspaper fell from my hand. Ben Smith was mopping near Minnie's bathroom. And now I knew why the nursing station was empty. They were all helping to strip Minnie's empty bed.

When my newspaper hit the floor, Miss Givens looked up. She quietly walked over and took my hand. "Miss Osbourne passed in her sleep," she said. "I came in to wake her and she was gone. I'm sorry," she added. "I know you were close."

I think I said thank you; I don't recall. I know I went back to my office and locked the door. Sitting at my desk, I propped my feet and leaned back. The empty chair was right in front of me.

I didn't cry that day. There were a few tears later and at times still, like now, when I think back on Minnie and me, a few tears yet, but all in all I just have firm, happy memories. I felt bad about not saying goodbye, but I'd dealt with death enough times to know that the package rarely gets wrapped neatly. There are always a few loose ends.

For a while I blamed myself for not being more sensitive to Minnie's decline toward the end, for being too concerned with meetings and numbers, but I think I've finally made my peace with that, too. What could I have done, really? She was an old woman who died in her sleep. For her to have lived meant enduring the empty, progressive agony of advancing Alzheimer's and the gradual loss, one by one, of all her precious memories.

I think things went about as well as could be expected. Minnie died doing what she liked best. She went in the middle of a good fight, a real rumble. She'd stood one final time on the right side. FDR would have been proud.

It was a while before I went back outside. Things being what they are at The Bin, by the time I hit the nursing station, someone new was checking into Minnie's room.

III

Minnie Osbourne was buried three days later at a public cemetery in a pauper's grave. I phoned her son to tell him of his mother's passing. When I asked about funeral plans he replied, "Doesn't the county make some provisions for that?" I had to bite my lip to keep from screaming.

Miss Givens, Dr. Ashwin, Nurse Wilson, and I attended the small service graciously provided by Miss Givens's local Baptist congregation. Besides the minister, we were the only people there. I spoke briefly, as did Miss Givens. Then we went to the cemetery.

Big Daddy Benson was reelected to his supervisor's seat but not by the usual wide margin of victory. He spent a little more time in the ghetto after that and, true to his word, the freeway plans were dropped. His proposal to raise our budget was also soundly defeated.

As I learned, when dealing with public mental health issues, most times it's a victory just to come out even.

My one hope from this struggle was that somehow, someway, some of those people eating behind some of those supermarkets, those people sleeping in doorways and culverts, those people shivering on sidewalk steam grills, could know they had a friend. That in their godforsaken, hellish world, a thin black lady from Louisiana had been on their side when it mattered.

IV

Minnie Osbourne's passing gave Thanksgiving that year a poignant, introspective quality. It made me see my life in a slightly different light. I reflected back on what was truly meaningful. I realized how grateful I was for my good parents, how I truly cherished my children, and how thankful I was that they were healthy. And most especially it made me appreciate my loving wife. I needed to be reminded of how blessed I was.

It may sound corny but knowing Minnie gave me a new respect for whatever you want to call The Indomitable Human Spirit. I also

94

found new meaning in the words pride, honor, and compassion. But most of all, I came to know how true nobility can be embodied in a human being. She was quite a lady.

I acted a little odd that weekend. My parents drove down from San Francisco and my wife's family flew in from Arizona. We had a big turkey and everything that went with it. I'd explained to my wife about Minnie, but somehow I don't think I accurately conveyed my true feelings. She thought I was acting strangely as well.

I remember spending more time than usual with my dad and being truly interested in what was happening in his life. I asked about his golf game. I asked about his friends. I asked how he was feeling about retirement.

This may be normal father-son stuff in most families, but until then it hadn't been in ours. As a rule, we'd always been a fairly tight-lipped group. I think my sudden interest in emotions and closeness caught my dad a little off guard. "Isn't there a game on?" he said about ten minutes into one conversation.

I spent time with my in-laws, making a special effort to speak with my wife's mother. I smiled. I inquired. We laughed. For the first time in a long while, maybe ever, we shared an uncombative moment. It all proved to be too much for her, too. "I think Linda needs help in the kitchen," she finally said, rising from the couch.

I've always been pretty close with my mom, so things between us went on pretty much as usual. I did, however, mention twice that I loved her, which drew an infinitesimally raised eyebrow.

My kids were the most open about their feelings. After carefully observing my behaviour all day, after I'd spent an uncomplaining hour watching them play Nintendo and agreeing to raise their allowance, they cornered their mother in the kitchen.

"Is Dad feeling alright?" I heard them ask.

I didn't hear my wife's reply.

V

As Dr. Ashwin had explained to me, empathy is a core concept in psychiatry. It's more than merely sympathizing with a patient's problems. It means truly feeling for them. Feeling with them. For some residents, especially those, like myself, who were first trained in other medical disciplines where lab tests, procedures, and scanners predominate, it's a hard concept to get the hang of. It doesn't come easily. I know in my case it didn't.

Empathy, as I see it, is understanding someone else's dilemma on a personal level. Obtaining it, for most, I think is like studying a foreign language. You struggle along for months or years until finally somehow you're fluent. From talking with residents at other hospitals, this seems to be the process.

At The Bin, of course, things rarely go like other places. We got our lesson in empathy in one fell swoop. I know I certainly learned to empathize with our patients' day-to-day struggles. I learned to connect. I learned what was really going on in my patients' lives.

I learned all that stuff real quick. I learned it during the two weeks I stayed in The Bin.

NINE

ABLE TO LEAP TALL BUILDINGS

I

COME THE FIRST of December we got a real treat on Ward Three. We were assigned an extra resident. Dr. Ashwin and I were delighted. This meant another man at the oars. Another pair of shoulders to heft the burden. When we got the news, we were almost giddy. We spoke rapidly and gestured with our hands. We envisioned time to read in the library. Thirty minutes for lunch. Going home before dark. None of this materialized, of course, but it made for one particularly pleasant morning.

This just wasn't any resident we were getting, either. This was Glen Charles, resident extraordinaire. I'd heard about Dr. Charles almost from the day I arrived at The Bin. He was a hospital legend.

Dr. Charles had grown up in the area, just a stone's throw, in fact, from County General. This was back before the cocaine era. Back before the door out of the ghetto was replaced by an enormous, drug-fueled, sucking sump drain. He'd starred academically during high school as well as garnering all-state honors on the football field. In my fantasy he'd dated the head cheerleader, too.

A scholarship to Yale followed with medical school at Cornell. Any residency program would have been honored to take him. We were grateful that he'd selected County General.

Dr. Charles, now in his last year of training, had already, it was rumored, received two lucrative offers to join private-practice groups. The previous year he'd published a well-received research paper while carrying his full clinical load. No doubt this cut into his social life with Lois Lane.

I was extremely anxious to meet him and I must admit more than a little curious. I'll see for myself, I said. We'll have to check this guy out in person was my public stance. I practiced acting cool and unimpressed. I promised myself I wasn't going to fawn like the rest of them. Truthfully, I was excited as hell when he walked through the door.

Dr. Singh left rounds to go out and meet Dr. Charles. That should have been my first clue. As we were all introduced, Miss Givens actually seemed coquettish. I mumbled something stupid and sat down. Dr. Glen Charles just had an effect on people.

My initial apprehension and thinly veiled jealousy faded that morning like so much snow in the sun. Tall with the still-sturdy build of a former running back, Glen Charles commanded your immediate attention. His smooth dark skin was unlined. You couldn't say he was classically handsome. He just had a presence. Almost like an aura. He put you in mind of naming your children after him.

At the conclusion of rounds that morning, I was also convinced that Dr. Charles knew more psychiatry than any man alive, at least any man alive that I knew. "I'm looking forward to working with you," Dr. Charles said, extending his hand as we stood in the hallway.

"Believe me, the pleasure's mine, Doctor Charles," I replied.

"Just Glen, please," he said with a warm smile.

"Sure, Glen," I said, smiling back. "All that and a nice guy, too," I thought, walking back to my office.

II

We all got along great that first week together on Ward Three. Listening to Drs. Singh, Ashwin, and Charles, I was really learning something. Each day I felt it stronger and stronger. I knew I was onto a good thing.

Until Miss Givens arrived one afternoon, that is. It was December tenth. She stormed into the nursing station, slamming the door so hard the windows shuddered. Two patients in the hall jumped like they'd been shot. "Those devious, cheap sons of bitches!" she boomed, swiping at a stack of progress notes with her hand. Paper filled the air like leaves. "Goddamned honky assholes," she fumed, whirling into her chair.

I took this as my cue to leave quietly.

Miss Givens had just returned from a Local 220 meeting. That was the county nursing and maintenance employee union. They'd been negotiating a new contract since August. The previous agreement was set to expire on the fourteenth, a mere four days away. The county, apparently, had promised a three-year deal and now, no doubt, expecting to prey on last minute rank-and-file disunity, they'd revoked the offer in favor of a two-year pact. Less money than originally planned was involved as well. Miss Givens was understandably irate. She was County General's union rep.

The issue of a county nurse's strike was very sticky business. First off, any time medical people strike, patients suffer and nobody wants that. For years management had played this guilt card skillfully and often. But as county pay scales slipped further and further below industry standards, enough apparently was enough.

Second was the racial thing. The entire county board was white. In contrast, the majority of their nurses and nearly all the maintenance crews were black.

The third issue was sort of an odd one. It was more of a philosophical point really. The main proponent of the idea was Supervisor Ronald Hadley. Hadley represented Pacific Palisades, an affluent area on the west side of town. His argument went like this: There are tens of thousands of homeless people in the county, of which roughly fifty percent are mentally ill. There are only 250 psychiatric beds in the entire county hospital system. If all the beds disappeared, would it really matter? What's another few hundred insane people when you're dealing with those kinds of numbers?

I have always wanted to meet Supervisor Hadley. I'm certain he's a very odd man. Thus, one final concern about a strike was that Hadley was right and it really wouldn't matter. Once closed, maybe the whole damn system would just stay that way.

I know very little about labor matters and even less about strike negotiations, but I got the strong sense that whatever the issues were in this particular battle, they'd finally gotten personal.

"That tight-assed jerk," Miss Givens seethed whenever Supervisor Hadley's name came up in casual conversation. "I'd like to see someone kick his white butt from here to Orange County." This or a very similar response was gotten every time any of the supervisors' names were brought up. She and the other nurses were hot and getting hotter.

As the strike deadline neared, things got downright ugly. "Hadley accuses local 220 rep of unfair tactics," the headline read one morning in the paper. It seems Miss Givens had bussed a group of our outpatients down to Hadley's office and paraded around out front with signs. By then Miss Givens had given up her tirades. Instead, she prowled the halls of Ward Three in total silence, her jaw clenched so tight it might as well have been wired.

Sadly, the county, it seemed, was preparing for the worst. Instead of further bargaining, they launched an all-out recruiting campaign for part-time nurses to fill the anticipated void. The salary being offered was extraordinary, which only served to infuriate our nurses further. "If they've got that kind of money to throw around," Miss Givens said quite correctly, I believe, "then why not dump it in the contract?" We had applicants from as far away as St. Louis.

With an impending strike, I had three patients that were special concerns. Mae Peterson, a middle-aged white woman in the tortuous throes of an abysmal depression, had come to us from the main hospital ER where they'd sutured two long lacerations on each of her forearms. She'd made them herself. Mae spoke only of blackness and despair. Suicide was a definite risk. She had to be watched around the clock.

Abdul Aziz was in the middle of his first manic break. A well-to-do rug merchant originally from Iran, Mr. Aziz had found his way to The Bin after abruptly leaving his downtown store one afternoon and drawing the majority of his family savings from the bank. He was arrested after showering the ghetto streets with bills from the window of his moving car. The sheriff estimated Mr. Aziz was traveling in excess of eighty miles an hour.

Despite my best efforts at medication, Mr. Aziz hadn't stopped yelling, singing, and pacing for the two days he'd been on the ward. I'd begun him on lithium, a potentially dangerous drug. He needed frequent blood levels to be drawn and monitored.

And then there was Ricky Myers. "So there's going to be a strike," he said during one of our obligatory meetings.

"That's what I hear," I replied. Then he smiled that smile I hated.

"Good," he said. "This place could use some excitement."

I had no idea who they were going to import to watch Ricky Myers. I often wished Supervisor Hadley could come down and spend some time with him, however.

Midnight, December fourteenth came and went. No settlement. No contract. No nurses.

III

"Good morning," I said to the befuddled-looking little white woman sitting in Miss Givens's nursing-station chair. It was eight o'clock on our first strike morning.

The woman startled and spun around. As if saying the pledge of allegiance, her right hand was on her heart. "What?" she stammered. "Who are you?"

"I'm Doctor Seager," I said in my best calm voice. "I'm an intern here at County General. I work on this ward."

"Thank God," the woman said with an audible sigh. "If one more patient comes barging in here, I . . . I . . . I don't know," she concluded, her breathing getting a little rapid again.

I read her name tag. "Miss Larkin," I said, gingerly touching her shoulder, "would you like to rest a while in my office?"

Just then Abdul Aziz went striding by. His arms were raised in the air. "I am God," he sang at the top of his voice. "I fuck God. You fuck God."

Miss Larkin began to backpedal in her chair. I think she was trying to jump into my lap.

"This way," I said, pointing to the door. "A little time out and things will look a lot better."

Miss Larkin looked over her shoulder five times as we walked down the hall. "The letter never said anything about this," she muttered again and again.

"Used to private hospital work are you?" I said, opening my office

102

door. Miss Larkin looked up and down the hall one last time before I left her. "Goddamn lunatics," she mumbled.

I saw Glen Charles and Anita Ashwin coming down the hall. "How are things?" Anita asked with a smile.

"Have you met Miss Larkin, our new charge nurse yet?" I asked.

"No," Drs. Charles and Ashwin said simultaneously.

"Well, if you need her," I said, nodding to my office door, "she's taking a little break. Seems she just discovered that all our patients are mentally ill."

That first week was a disaster. Miss Larkin spent more time in my office than I did. I felt sorry for her. I remembered when I'd first come to The Bin. I was pretty sure the county's recruiting ad promising all that money had neglected to mention a detail or two.

To make matters worse, Miss Larkin was also the only nurse assigned to our ward on the day shift. Other people had come, taken one look at the place, and turned right around. For the duration of the strike it looked like this was all the nursing help we were going to get.

Miss Larkin had spent the last ten years at a desk job and came to County General, she said, "to brush up on my clinical skills." The poor woman just had no clue. In the space of five days, three patients got the wrong medication, I found a sharp-edged comb in Mae Peterson's room, beds went unchanged, and our paperwork was hopelessly behind. By week's end, my considerable well of patience was running very low. We were foundering badly.

The capper, however, came when I arrived at work that Friday. As I walked in the door I could instantly feel the change. It was quiet. And Miss Larkin was actually in the nursing station where she seemed to be working. Smiling and signing, she was transferring papers from a large stack on her left to a small pile on her right.

"Good morning, Doctor Seager," she said brightly. "Can I get you some coffee?" She set down her pen.

"No, thanks," I said, staring around in amazement. By then Glen Charles was coming through the door. He looked confused as well.

"What's wrong with this picture?" he said, staring first at Miss Larkin, then out into the serene, empty corridors.

"Miss Larkin," I said hesitantly, "where are the patients?"

"They're all in restraints," she replied proudly. "Why didn't you tell me about this restraint business before? We could have avoided all those problems. Now," she added confidently, "we can finally get some work done."

IV

We barely had the time and manpower to release everyone before Dr. Singh arrived, but, fortunately, we made it. I'd only seen him angry once before and I knew Miss Larkin didn't need that. She was teetering on the edge as it was.

After an hour of uncomfortably disorganized rounds, Dr. Ashwin, Dr. Charles, and I had an emergency meeting in Dr. Ashwin's office. There was no end in sight to the strike; in fact, it seemed, if the papers were to be believed, things had only become more acrimonious. And, to be honest, with no new patients being admitted to any county psych facility, mental illness had not run rampant on the streets. Not much, really, on the outside had changed at all.

But the outside was not our concern. We had to do something about Ward Three and do it now. It was a dispirited group of doctors that gathered that day.

"Maybe we could take up a collection and bribe Miss Givens to come back," Dr. Charles said, and I wasn't sure if he was joking.

"May God strike me dead if I ever utter an unkind word about that woman," I said.

We heard patients milling around in the hall and just as quickly we heard Miss Larkin's quick, crisp steps going by and the door to my office open and close.

"Well, gentlemen?" Dr. Ashwin said with a smile.

We came up with the only plan we could. None of us liked it but all agreed there was simply no other way. It meant missing time with our families. It probably meant missing Christmas at home as well. It probably meant many things, none of which could have been foreseen at that little get-together.

Our plan was to move onto Ward Three until the strike was over. So beginning that same night, that's what we did. I called my wife right after the meeting broke up and explained our predicament along with the proposed solution. After a short pause she said she understood. "It should only be for a few days," I added brightly. Then there was a longer pause.

"I'm sure you're right," Linda replied. I could hear the kids clamoring in the background.

TEN

HITTING THE WALL

I

"BEN," I called out toward the light coming from behind the old boiler. "Ben, I need your help."

"Yes, sir, Doctor Seager," Ben said. "Over here."

As I stepped into Ben Smith's small hideout, he stood from his bed and closed the book he'd been reading. He looked nervous. "I'm not in any trouble, am I, sir?" Ben asked straight off.

I always had trouble with Ben Smith calling me "sir." It made me distinctly uncomfortable and yet, somehow, I could never bring myself to ask him to stop. Whenever I saw Ben, or almost any older black person, I couldn't help but remember all the television and magazine images I'd seen while growing up. The pictures of the marches and the firehoses and bombed-out churches and lynchings and a fat white sheriff chewing Red Man tobacco.

I guess it was a combination of guilt, remorse, and respect. I figured after enough time had passed this feeling would subside. But it never did. Which, I suppose, if you think about it, is probably just as well.

"No, Ben, there's no trouble," I said. "I need your help."

Ben looked visibly relieved. He'd faced a real problem when Local 220 went on strike. All our maintenance crews belonged to the same union as the nurses, so technically Ben Smith was on strike, too. This meant he now had to spend all his days as well as nights in the basement. And during the day there were people around. His anxiety was understandable.

I explained to Ben that while the county had managed to find some replacement nurses, they hadn't bothered to locate new custodial men. The trash was beginning to pile up and the floors looked like hell. We had, I said, decided to take matters into our own hands. I was downstairs asking Ben where he kept his supplies and how to work his bucket.

Ben seemed apprehensive again but he told me what I needed to know. "You be careful, sir," he said finally.

I was touched by Ben's concern. "Don't worry, I won't get hurt," I said with a smile.

"I truly hope not, sir," Ben replied. "But I was talking about my mop and bucket."

"I'll be careful, Ben," I said and nodded.

II

Those first few days had kind of a larklike quality to them. The feeling you get when you're in a tough situation and handling things pretty well. It was an adventure.

Dr. Charles, Dr. Ashwin, and I quickly set up a routine. Our days were pretty much the same; after all we were still the doctors in charge of the place. After the day crew left, however, we swung into action.

I began by giving the hallway and nursing station a good mopping.

While initially Ben's bucket and wringer were a bit unwieldy, in no time I pretty much had the hang of it. Soon I was swishing and rinsing like a pro.

While I cleaned the linoleum, Dr. Charles took care of the trash, emptying all the little basket liners into big plastic leaf bags, which he hauled down to the dumpsters out back. He did the light dusting as well. Anita and the lone replacement nurse, Emma Fernandez, a slender wisp of a Filipino woman who, as best we could guess, spoke ten words of English, saw to the patients' meals and medications. Together, as a final chore, we all cleaned the bathrooms.

The patients' reaction to this was very interesting. At first they were amused, standing in small groups outside the nursing station and chuckling as I mopped. When I was done, without fail, someone would point down to the floor and mouth, "Missed a spot." When we did a bathroom, each patient couldn't help poking his head in three or four times just to be certain he was seeing what he thought he was seeing.

Then a strange thing happened. "Let me help you," Mae Peterson said, taking a rag from my bucket. I'd just finished soaping her bathroom floor. "Mirrors are a pain. I should know. I've done enough of them." As she spritzed Windex on the glass above her sink, I realized this was the first time I'd seen her out of bed in a week.

"Where did you do all those mirrors?" I said, swinging my mop around to do a corner.

Mae smiled a sad smile. "It's a long story," she said.

"I've got all night," I replied.

And so we began to talk. Not in any classical "dynamic" type way that I'd been reading so much about and struggling to master. We talked as friends, as two human beings who just happened to be cleaning a bathroom at the time. It was, in looking back, my first experience with true therapy, both for Mae and for me.

Mae had done all those windows and mirrors because as a young

109

woman—she was now fifty-six—she'd fallen in love with an aspiring attorney. They married and after he became a partner in his law firm, the couple moved to the exclusive Palos Verdes section of town. Into, apparently, a house with lots of windows and mirrors to clean.

"Any children?" I asked and Mae brightened. She motioned for me to follow her into her room. From a nightstand drawer she produced a dog-eared snapshot of two grinning teenage boys with hair a little too short and ears a little too big. Judging from a car parked in the background, the year was 1975.

"Nice-looking kids," I said, turning the photo up a bit to get better light. "What are they doing now?"

Again Mae smiled. "Bob, the oldest, is a pilot for the Navy or 'aviator' as I guess they like to be called," she said proudly. "And Mike's an accountant. They live back East somewhere."

It was that last sentence that got me. It was one I'd heard all too often since coming to County General. Where once a young couple with two strapping sons had happily taken a Polaroid in front of their stunning house, now Mae Peterson was showing me old pictures of people who lived "back East somewhere" as we prepared to finish cleaning her bathroom at County General, The Bin, the last stop on the rail line.

Like I said, this was a story I heard with regularity. Our patients weren't born street people or transients or bums or whatever you want to call them. Many had once lived lives exactly like you and I. They'd owned homes, paid taxes, had weddings. They have children and parents. They once had hopes and plans for the future just like us.

But something got in the way of those hopes and plans. These people came down with mental illness, the modern leprosy.

Mae Peterson, like most of our patients, was a victim of what's called the "drift down theory". Back in the forties and fifties when people decided to finally look into mental illness, the fact that a lot more sick people lived in the ghetto than in the suburbs was surprising. The question was this: Did poverty make you mentally ill or did these people "drift down" from somewhere else? The drift down theory won out.

Mae Peterson had, admittedly, drifted quite a ways, but her story was not unique. Many of our ragged, urine-stained patients had degrees from prestigious universities. Some had worn suits and ties at jobs with companies whose names you would instantly recognize. They've traded stock and managed banks. Some had, no doubt, obliviously driven past the street people of their day, too, the people they would themselves someday become.

Mae's form of mental leprosy was depression. It started, she said, in her early thirties. "It was like a black hole opened up," she said. "And I fell in."

I doubt if many of us know what it means to be truly depressed. Not to be "sad" or "down" or "blue," but to be depressed. To know real despair. To feel absolutely hopeless. To honestly believe that you're completely worthless and deserving of the torture you are forced to endure.

"My husband put up with me as long as he could," Mae said as she sat on the side of the bed and I rested on a window ledge. "He wasn't a bad man. Who wants a wife that spends half the year in bed sobbing?"

Mae lost her house in the divorce and the drift had begun. Her children soon went off to college. "I was in bad shape. I didn't visit very often," she said sadly. "Then we just sort of lost contact."

That's when Mae first tried to end her life. When she first held out her wrist to a razor and sliced flesh.

"My sister took me in when I got out of the hospital," Mae said. "But she had a family of her own to raise and she worked. For about a year things were fine. Then I got sick again."

This time after another hospital stay Mae rented an apartment by herself. Drift. She tried to hold a job but couldn't. Drift. She was evicted. Drift. Alimony checks stopped coming. Drift. She applied for public relief. Drift. A move to a board-and-care home. Drift. A razor once again to the arm. The Bin.

I'll give you my spiel on depression just as I give it to all my depressed patients, just as I gave it to Mae Peterson that night.

"Depression is not a moral failure. It's not something over which you have control. You cannot say, 'If only I had been a stronger and better person this wouldn't have happened.' You're not to blame. You are not being punished. You don't deserve this.

"Depression is a biochemical disease of the brain just like diabetes is a biochemical disease of the body. And just as diabetics need insulin, you will require medication as well.

"I can't guarantee anything, but I believe and I want you to believe that you're going to feel better. And, hopefully, stay better."

Mae Peterson and I never got around to finishing the bathroom that night. We spent the evening simply talking. When I left it was nearly ten. And Mae had something resembling a smile on her face. The whole experience was a revelation.

III

The one routine that wasn't disrupted by the strike, the one routine we still had to follow, was night call. The novelty of working all night had quickly worn off and with all the added pressure we were under anyway, it was just an additional burden. But it had to be done, so we continued to do it. As I walked over to the PES to begin my shift that late December evening, I wasn't in the best frame of mind.

I should have known my mood wasn't going to improve when I saw Drs. Jones and Phillips, the pair that Dr. Ashwin and I were coming to relieve. As we walked into the small office they were both slumped in their chairs, their eyes slightly glazed. They looked, in fact, like they'd both been struck with baseball bats. At the sight of fresh troops, however, they brightened. Dr. Jones had a slightly malicious grin on his face.

"Welcome," he said, sitting straight. "Can I get you anything? Coffee? Tea? Cyanide?"

"That bad?" I said and my heart sank further.

Dr. Jones pointed to the two-page patient roster he held in his hand. "Thirty-two big ones," he said with that same devilish grin.

"That's impossible," Dr. Ashwin sputtered. "We only have twelve beds."

"We're very inventive down here," Dr. Phillips said, gesturing out toward the large dayroom. The floor was completely covered with army cots. "We called the National Guard armory," Phillips added. "They were only too glad to help."

I thought we'd been under undue strain up on Ward Three because of the strike, but suddenly I knew it was probably nothing compared to Phillips and Jones's job in the PES. The place looked like a refugee camp.

It took nearly an hour just to get through the list of names, and with all the talk about diagnoses, medications, legal status, physical diseases, allergies, etc., after a while everything just seemed like a hopeless jumble.

Jones and Phillips looked euphoric when they finally stood to leave. But their faces dropped again when Dr. Ashwin said, "See you in the morning."

Finally it was just me and Dr. Ashwin against a sea of ailing humanity. "I feel a little fever coming on," Anita said, lightly touching the back of her hand to her forehead. "Why don't you clean things up down here while I go lie down. I'll check back around midnight." That was the last laugh we'd share for some time.

With Christmas only a few days away, I know the season had

something to do with it. And I hadn't been home in days. And I was sick of eating county food. And I knew I'd be up all night. It was lots of things. Some of which were, perhaps, understandable. But even given that, there was still no excuse for my behaviour. I just lost it.

Dr. Ashwin and I divided the work as best we could. She stayed downstairs to sort through the throng of people entrusted to our care while I went upstairs to man the triage desk. It didn't help to find the waiting room jammed.

Things went as well as could be expected for a while. With all the practice I'd gotten taking night call for the past six months, it was getting easier for me to spot homeless people pretending to be mentally ill. I'd picked up a few tips along the way from the older residents, like checking under a person's seat for bundled clothing or a suitcase. Or confronting them with the issue right off. "Are you looking for a place to stay?" I'd ask before they'd gotten a chance to even start their recitation about voices, strange beliefs, and suicide. The true mentally ill took the question in stride. "No," they'd reply simply and then give me the name of their board-and-care home. The others were always taken aback for just a second and that was that.

As I said, I detested my job as gatekeeper for the homeless and, good at it or not, it was still a painful task sending people back into the night. So after hustling my fifth person out the door, I was not in top shape. And then it was just the wrong person coming at the wrong time. Or whatever. But things went straight downhill from there.

I'd just settled across the desk from a new patient when the front doors slid open and two policemen led in a handcuffed man. "I'm Jesus," the man was muttering. "Kill me. I'm Jesus."

My heart sank when I saw the man's face. I knew Slick Eddie James only too well. I knew the story the cops were going to tell me. I knew they were going to place him on a hold, which meant squeezing in another cot downstairs. And I knew I faced a mound of unnecessary paperwork.

Slick Eddie James was a thief. Nothing major, mainly small-time stuff—car batteries, hub caps, wallets, that kind of thing. "Gotta keep under that grand larceny rap," he'd explained to me the last time he'd been in.

Eddie had the system pegged perfectly. He knew with the volume of work he did, arrests were an occupational hazard. He also knew how much policemen detested busy work, especially for the petty stuff he was stealing. Finally, he knew there was an acceptable way for him to relieve the cops of that hated chore.

"We caught him jacking open the hood of a car," one officer said with a straight face. "On the way to the station he started saying all this crazy stuff about Jesus, so I thought you'd better check him out."

I looked at Eddie. I looked at the two cops. I looked at my waiting room full of patients. Then I just started shouting.

I screamed at Slick Eddie. I screamed at the cops. I even screamed at the poor sign-in clerk who only filled out the charts. I let everyone know my feelings about the homeless and the county board of supervisors and about people who manipulate the system.

I emphasized my displeasure with criminals and drug addicts always trying to get into the hospital while the courts kept letting the truly mentally ill out. I think I mentioned my wife and kids. I said how tired I was.

After covering all my topics pretty well, I stopped. My face was flushed, my hands shaking. When I glanced around, everyone in the waiting room was staring at me. Security guards were staring at me, as were the two cops and receptionist. Slick Eddie had a smile on his face.

I felt like an idiot. "I'm sorry," I said once I'd come back to my senses. "I don't know what came over me."

I expected the others to vent their anger at me in return and I would have deserved it. But, strangely, they all took my outburst in stride. The secretary went back to her computer. The cops started filling out their hold forms. And everyone in the waiting room sat back down again.

Noting my confusion, one of the security guards took me aside. "Don't worry, Doc," he said. "Happens to everyone before they leave here. In fact we were all a little surprised it took you this long to go off."

All I could do was shake my head.

"Would you like me to take the patient down now?" the guard added.

ELEVEN

LIVING WITH THE FORGOTTEN

I

I'D LIKE TO SAY that my wife and kids took this strike business pretty well. They did their best, but I know they hated it. "You realize your parents are coming for Christmas Eve," my wife said when I finally spent a night at home, as Dr. Charles, Dr. Ashwin, and I had decided it was best for all of us to do in rotation. She was folding a basket of towels fresh from the dryer. She wasn't looking at me.

"Yes, I know," I replied wearily. I knew she knew I knew. Then she went on silently folding.

My youngest son was more to the point. "What kind of stupid job do you have, anyway?" he said as I walked through the door that first night back. I'd been wondering the same thing myself.

By the next morning things had turned openly hostile. "Goodbye," I said, standing from the breakfast table. "You have a good day at school."

All three kids looked at me with thinly veiled contempt. "We're on vacation, Dad," my daughter said.

"You know, for Christmas," my oldest boy added.

"When families are supposed to be together," my youngest son concluded.

My wife met me at the door. "What you're doing is important," she said, taking my hand. "It's just hard for them to understand. It's a little hard for me to understand sometimes too."

I wasn't certain I understood much of anything either, but I tried to leave on a cheerful note. "Hang in there," I said. "This thing can't go on much longer." Then I gave her a kiss and left.

At work I unfolded the newspaper I'd tucked under my arm. "County breaks off talks with nurses," the main story said. It was December twenty-first.

II

Since I'd taken up as a live-in doctor, I noticed a subtle shift in my feelings about Ward Three. I first noticed the change at night.

I'd previously thought of our ward as a fairly nice place, as county psychiatric facilities went. I'd arrive in the morning feeling good. The staff was pleasant. Rounds were stimulating. And with the exception of Ricky Myers, I'd found something to enjoy in all my patients. I'd always felt safe. But then I got to go home in the evening.

Spending all those nights on the ward, however, altered things. I began to sense with clear and ever-increasing clarity, exactly why my patients were so anxious to get out of there.

I think it started with the door—my first fear. It's big and made of heavy metal. It gives a real prison-cell clang when it shuts. But the main thing is it's locked.

There is something so claustrophobically eerie about that. At night, when you're lying in bed and you hear that big jolt, it makes the hair on the back of your neck stand up.

I felt that way and I had a set of keys in my pants pocket. What must the patients have been feeling?

My second fear, which I recognized as somewhat deeper and more irrational, was that, despite having my keys and being an employee of The Bin, maybe *I'd* never get out of there because of some foul up no matter how far fetched or remote. It was a fear I did, and do, find difficult to articulate. But now I understand why any delay, be it only hours, in my patients' discharge times, caused them so much anxiety. You just never know.

My third fear was grounded somewhat more firmly in reality. When you're locked up with Ricky Myers, I think a certain amount of apprehension can be expected. I think Minnie Osbourne summed it up best. One day early in our conversations she seemed strangely troubled. "There's a dark evil inside someone here," she said, her failing eyes narrowing. "I feel it when I'm out on the ward as strongly as I feel you here with me now."

I didn't know what to say. "I'm sure . . ." I began finally, but she cut me off.

"Believe me," Minnie said firmly. "You're in for a bad happening."

That was Ricky Myers. He felt like a bad happening.

Darkness in and of itself had a lot to do with my problems. It's a regressive, disorienting phenomenon at best. And these are two qualities for mental patients that don't necessarily serve their best interests. At night the lid gets a little loose. Things normally contained tend to seep out.

People scream. There are footsteps and peels of laughter. You hear distant noises that defy classification. It's a wonder anyone gets any sleep at all. I kept one eye open the whole time I was there.

III

In an effort to limit confusion during the strike, the hospital had decided to close its doors to all but the most extreme emergency admissions. For Drs. Charles, Ashwin, and me this was a real blessing. It gave us something we rarely had on Ward Three—a stable population.

A stable population meant a chance to know our patients better and for me, in particular, it was a chance to get to know a couple of people real well, or at least so I thought at the time. One of these people was Glen Charles. We talked a lot. What I learned from our discussions would explain a great deal about what happened later. The other person I got to know was Ricky Myers.

As I said, it took the patients awhile to adjust to us being on the ward at night. I don't think they knew quite what to make of the whole thing. We had trouble relating.

What finally broke the ice, however, was Pat Sajak and his stupid "Wheel of Fortune." The patients loved that program. It was a real common denominator. The most loosely wrapped people were glued to the set while Vanna White flipped those letters and contestants bid for outrageously priced "gift items." Even Mr. Aziz stopped pacing and singing a little when Wheel came on.

I detested the show but bowed to the will of the majority. It came on just as dinner trays were arriving and there was only the lone TV set. One night after I'd returned from my one evening at home, a particularly difficult puzzle came up. Those people around the wheel spun so many times I began to get dizzy. Then the fools kept calling for used letters. One man asked for an *R* three times in a row. The audience and our dinner crowd thought it was hilarious. From the look on his face, Pat Sajak felt about the same way I did.

All the patients and Dr. Charles and I were guessing at the puzzle but to no avail. Then a voice came from the back of the room.

"To thine own self be true," someone said.

"Of course," Dr. Charles shouted immediately.

We turned around. The voice belonged to Ricky Myers. No doubt he sensed the surprise in our expressions. "It's from Shakespeare," he said curtly. "Laertes' speech to Hamlet." Then he turned to leave. "I'm not stupid," he added, disappearing out the door.

That little exchange gave me the strangest feeling. I was confused, a bit angry, and more than a little ashamed of myself. In six months as Myers's doctor that was the first contact we'd had that could even remotely be labeled as human.

His last sentence was what got me: "I'm not stupid." I suddenly realized that I didn't know Myers wasn't stupid. I didn't know whether he was or wasn't anything. Other than a list of his crimes, I didn't know anything about him at all.

Did I want to know? Do monsters deserve therapy? What unconscious fears did Myers rouse in me that made me behave toward him the way I did? I think Dr. Charles was having some of the same thoughts.

"I'm glad he's your patient," he said as we returned to dinner.

IV

Fortunately, it was a relatively quiet night. After the patients went to bed, Dr. Charles and I had a chance to sit down. It was a real eye-opener for me. I guess it's always strange getting to know your heroes personally.

The conversation began casually enough. We were alone in the dayroom staring blankly at a TV program neither of us wanted to watch. It was Dr. Charles who finally stood and turned off the sound.

"Do you mind?" he said, reaching for the knob. "I get so tired of this drivel all day long."

The quiet was a welcome relief. I picked up a section of newspaper from a nearby table and began to read.

"You play gin rummy?" Dr. Charles asked.

"Not well," I replied. "But I don't mind getting beat a few games."

So we played gin rummy and I got beat more than a few times. I don't think the man misplayed a card. As we shuffled and dealt we naturally began to talk.

"I understand you were quite the football star in school," I said after we'd played a hand.

"I guess so," Dr. Charles said with an odd smile.

"All-state tailback from what I hear," I said.

Dr. Charles got strangely quiet for a moment. "I haven't thought about high school in a long time," he said slowly, sort of looking past me. "I really hated that game," he added.

I remember how struck I was by that comment. It hinted at so much more.

We talked well into the night, long after the cards were stacked and put aside. We talked about two different childhoods. I told him about growing up in Utah under the shadow of the Wasatch mountains. He told me about the ghetto. I said what I remembered most was my team winning the city baseball championship when I was ten. Glen Charles told me about getting shot when he was fourteen.

We talked about fathers and how much it meant to us to please them. But the tone in our voices was different. As Dr. Charles spoke, I got the sense that he was saying, "I couldn't please him no matter what I did." "That man did love football," I remember him stating.

I talked about being just another kid at a rural California university. Glen Charles talked about being the only black person in his entire dorm building. We talked about grades and dating. I said I'd gone to medical school mainly to keep from going to Vietnam. Dr. Charles said not going to medical school had never been an option.

I said how hard medical school had been for me. I told him about my long hours with the books. I said I guessed I'd ranked somewhere in the middle of my class. Then I learned what truly long hours you have to endure to graduate at the top.

I told Glen a little bit about my wife and kids. "Someday I'll have to make time for that," he said, then changed the subject.

The last thing we talked about was success. Then I learned something else. I learned the difference between wanting something and being driven to it.

V

Until I did my extended stint on Ward Three I never realized how hard nurses work. During my ER years I guess I'd just been too busy to notice. And when I continued on with psychiatry, I just carried this same oblivious mind-set with me.

As a doctor you're used to ordering things—a form to be signed, a blood test drawn or an X ray taken—and just having them get done. It was a process I never took for granted again.

I got my lesson in who does what and how from Mr. Aziz, the rug merchant turned street philanthropist.

Mr. Aziz suffered from bipolar disorder, or what used to be called manic depression. In the official psychiatric classification book, *The American Psychiatric Association: Diagnostic and Statistical Manual of Mental Disorders,* third Edition, revised, or DSM-III-R for short (a handbook that lists all known psychiatric diagnoses and gives them each a number), bipolar disorder comes under the heading of "mood disorders." And is it ever.

"Bipolars," as they are called, suffer from either too much mood or not enough and often, in a periodic, predictable way, will swing, or cycle, between the two extremes—mania and depression. It's a rhythmic disease. Sort of like the coming and going of the tides or the regular changing of seasons.

Mr. Aziz had begun his disease process with a manic swing. Mania is not just feeling good. It's not just being happy. It's more than being unusually active. Mania begins with euphoria, passes through believing you're a billionaire, and lands when your thoughts are racing so fast your mouth can't catch up. It means not sleeping for a week or walking thirty-five miles to get a pack of cigarettes.

It can be a ruinous disease as Mr. Aziz would soon find out. During a manic break, normal, church-going people will suddenly buy six cars or fly around the world or have sex with a dozen people a night. They run up unbelievable debts and start lots of bar fights. When things finally settle down, generally due to medication, there is suddenly the piper to pay. Notes from MasterCard arrive asking how you plan to handle that $200,000 balance. The risk, of course, when these people get depressed, is that they'll take a gun to their head.

The mainstay treatment for bipolar disorder is lithium. Lithium, like sodium, is a natural element. Unlike sodium, however, it has, for reasons unknown, a mood-stabilizing effect. A famous California health spa, so the story goes, known for producing peace and tranquility in its patrons, was closed by the board of health when lithium was discovered in its therapeutic waters.

There are, unfortunately, problems with lithium. It's not a benign medication by any stretch. Too little does nothing. Too much can kill you. So for each patient a safe, effective middle ground must be found. And the only way to do this is to monitor blood levels. And the only way this gets done is to draw lots of blood from the person's arm. In order to do this, however, you have to catch them first.

It's a difficult proposition getting someone who believes they're omnipotent to submit to any request, let alone one that involves a painful needle. In Mr. Aziz's case, he was convinced that his vast wealth could buy him health. He wanted no part of the Ward Three staff or "peasants," as he called us.

Every day it was a monumental task getting his blood taken. We tried coaxing, pleading, begging, offering small rewards, but never with any success. Things always devolved into a wild chase down the hall, a frantic scramble, and finally restraints. Dr. Charles and I always ended up sweaty and angry.

Then we'd think of our regular diminutive nurses and all the lithium levels we'd ordered in the past.

"How in the hell do they do it?" I asked with amazement and admiration.

Dr. Charles shook his head. "I think they just make up the numbers and write them on the slips," he said.

"Who's ordering all this damned blood work anyway?" I said as we sat in the dayroom to catch our breath.

Dr. Charles only smiled.

TWELVE

'TIS THE SEASON TO BE LONELY

I

I MANAGED TO SPEND Christmas Eve at home with my family, which kept their anger and frustration levels temporarily below the boiling point. After some initial friction and bickering, the evening went rather well. We each opened a gift (surprise: Dad got a tie), we ate oyster stew, then everyone sat single file across the couch, feet perched on the coffee table, as we bathed in the inexplicably colorized light of "It's a Wonderful Life." Our evening was tinged, somewhat, however, by the fact that everyone knew that when Santa arrived in the morning and the turkey got carved tomorrow afternoon, I wouldn't be there.

Understandably, I wasn't in the best frame of mind to begin my Christmas Day on Ward Three. I was hoping that something during the day would cheer me up. Nothing did.

I wasn't sure what Christmas would be like on the ward, but certainly I thought there would be visitors, maybe some gifts, perhaps a few songs and laughs, the usual things I'd always assumed go along with Christmas even when you're ill. That, of course, was before I remembered.

What I'd neglected to consider was my basic premise concerning the mentally ill. I'd forgotten that no one cares about them. Not on Christmas. Not ever. And during the holidays, I learned, even the most out-of-touch patients somehow seemed to sense this. I can't imagine their despair.

Hardly anyone came out of their room the entire day, even for meals. The hallways echoed like tombs. No one came to visit. We didn't even get a phone call. Nothing. It was the longest day I'd ever spent. Dr. Charles and I barely spoke. Anita Ashwin was home for the day. Football droned endlessly from the dayroom TV. Needless to say, no one sang. No one laughed.

In mid-afternoon the spell was momentarily broken. I heard footsteps in the hallway but was too depressed to turn and look.

"Who do you like, Texas or Oklahoma?" the voice asked from behind me.

Now I didn't have to turn around. I knew it was Ricky Myers.

Strangely, surprisingly, gratefully, for the first time since I'd known him, I didn't feel like ice was running down my spine. I didn't know what I felt, but at least it wasn't fear. "Oklahoma," I managed to mumble.

And Myers looked different, too. The Manson glint and suspicious stare were gone. The vigilant posture had disappeared as well. For the first time, Ricky Myers didn't look like what he'd become, a crazed mass murderer, but what he'd once been, the third son of a garage mechanic from Salem, Oregon.

"A Sooner fan, huh?" Ricky said, still standing. For a change he seemed to be the uncomfortable one. I motioned to the chair beside me and Myers sat.

"You like football?" I asked after a prolonged silence.

Myers shook his head in an odd, jerky way. "I followed sports some when I was a kid," he said, "but then . . . well, I got away from it."

128

We sat quietly again for what seemed like an hour. I was pretending to watch the game. I noticed my foot was tapping. Finally Myers got right to the heart of things.

"You can ask me if you want," he said flatly, his eyes aimed straight ahead.

"Ask what?" I fumbled. I was suddenly so tense I could barely move.

Myers paused. "You can ask me why I did it," he said finally. "Why I killed all those people."

I can't really say Ricky Myers and I had a conversation that Christmas Day. I was much too unsettled for that and, frankly, I think Myers was too. It had been so long since anyone had actually spoken with him, someone who wasn't battling their own terror and hatred, I think he'd simply forgotten how to talk to people. And, in all fairness, he was the first mass murderer I'd met.

Myers's mannerisms were awkward, his inflections a bit off. He twitched when he moved his hands. I wasn't much better. We were both on an unmapped road.

Basically, I asked questions and Myers answered them. He'd first heard voices when he was fifteen. He was initially hospitalized a year later. His mother died when he was young. His father was an auto mechanic. He had an uncle with schizophrenia. He did okay in school. "I liked English," Myers said with something resembling a smile.

"Any girlfriends?" I asked.

This was the strangest moment of our "conversation." I thought I saw a flicker of sadness pass across Myers's face. "Had a wife once," he said, then waited a moment. "A baby, too. A boy."

"Congratulations," I said for lack of anything better. Myers didn't respond.

We talked another minute or two before our communal anxiety overwhelmed us. We made an excuse to break off and Myers went back to his room.

It took a while to collect my thoughts and impressions. Finally, I concluded, I didn't know what to make of it all. I was sure of one thing however. Myers wasn't hearing voices any more. He'd said so twice. He'd finally been on enough of the right medication and they'd slowly gone away. The voices, he said, were what made him kill.

Then I was struck with a chilling thought. Was I actually feeling a little sorry for the man? Was I proud of the job I'd done making his voices disappear? Did I think I'd somehow cured him? It was like someone slapped me in the face when I realized that's how Myers had gotten released from the last hospital, back when two young girls were still alive. Just the thought of falling into the same trap made me sick to my stomach. For the first time in years I knew what it felt like to need a drink.

II

Just after ten that night, after I'd called home and gotten a report on all the holiday happenings at my house, which only served to depress me further, after our nightly battle to draw Mr. Aziz's blood, after everything was quiet and only Dr. Charles and I were left in the dayroom, I saw Mae Peterson coming toward me from the hallway. She had a small package in her hand. It had been carefully wrapped in newsprint. Her hair was combed. She smiled at me.

"Merry Christmas," she said, handing me the gift.

I was so touched the words simply wouldn't come. So I unwrapped the present. It was a threadbare jewelry box.

"I don't understand," I finally managed to say.

"Open it," Mae said quietly.

I gently pried up the lid. Inside was a man's pocket watch. It was obviously very old and had seen many years of service. The hands were stopped at two-thirty. There was a small crack in the thick, faded crystal.

"It belonged to my father," Mae said as I lifted the old timepiece from its case. "He was a railroad man."

"But Mae . . ." I began and then stopped. I was going to say how I couldn't possibly accept the gift. How moved I was by the gesture. How the watch should go to someone in her family. But I didn't say any of it. I just held the watch in my hand. It was something about the look in Mae's eyes. It was a look of quiet happiness.

"But I have nothing for you," I said and Mae smiled again.

"What you gave me is worth more than a conductor's watch," she said, and I remembered the night we'd spent all those hours talking in her room.

"Merry Christmas, Mae Peterson," I said and gave her hug.

"Merry Christmas, Doctor Seager," Mae said, hugging me back.

III

That next morning Dr. Charles and I were first to arrive for rounds. We slid our chairs out from the large conference table and didn't really sit in them so much as we collapsed in them.

"If we have to stay here through New Year's," Dr. Charles said, folding his arms on the tabletop and laying his forehead on the back of his hands, "I'll bet your wife is going to shoot you."

"If we have to stay here through New Year's," I sighed, "I'll shoot myself."

And then it was over. Dr. Lamb, the psychologist, burst through the door. "The nurses are coming back," he said, spreading the morning paper in front of Dr. Charles and me.

I thought he was joking until I realized no one was that stupid. Glen

Charles and I were desperate men—and he'd been a football player. Then I saw the picture. Right there, big as life, both grinning wide as you please, were our Miss Givens and Supervisor Hadley. They were shaking hands. "Rare holiday session brings accord," the headline read. "Rank and file to vote today on new pact."

I showed the picture to Dr. Charles. "Thank God," he said and laid his head back down. Inside of a minute he was fast asleep.

IV

It happened the instant I set foot on Ward Three the next morning. "Medication!" Miss Givens boomed out into the hall through the half-open Dutch door of the nursing station. It was the sweetest sound I'd ever heard.

And judging from the patients' reaction, they were just as glad to have her back as I was. Instead of somberly forming a haphazard line to get their pills, they crowded around the door in bunches. You'd have thought we were giving away money.

"Boy, am I ever glad to see you," I said as I walked through the other nursing station door.

Miss Givens had just handed the last patient his medication and little juice cup. "Who's responsible for the mess this place is in?" she said without turning her head. "My files are so screwed up I can't find anything." She brushed past me. "No patient logs. Missing lab slips." She was scavenging the top of her desk. "And that dayroom. Have you seen the dayroom? Did the circus come through here while I was gone?"

Miss Givens went by me going the other way and headed out the door. "Where's Ben Smith?" she said from the hall. "He'd better get his lazy butt . . ." I didn't hear any more because Miss Givens disappeared into the dayroom.

I saw Andy Loar, one of Dr. Ashwin's patients, standing in the hall. A tiny black man in his sixties, he'd been on Ward Three for months. He'd been listening to Miss Givens, too. "Great to have her back," he said with a beaming smile.

"Isn't it," I agreed.

All things considered, it took surprisingly little time for things on the ward to return to normal. Ben Smith came back that first post-strike morning and was his usual pleasant, efficient self. I thanked him for the use of his equipment. "Floors never looked better," he said, but he was just being polite. Every time I saw him that day he was going from room to room shaking his head.

Miss Larkin dropped in briefly to collect her things. Crisp and smiling, she looked like a woman who'd just had a car lifted off her foot. "It was awfully pleasant working with you, Doctor Seager," she said, shaking my hand. "Now if I could just speak to Miss Givens for a moment, I'll be on my way."

"That's probably not the best idea," I said, gently prodding the woman toward the exit. "She's real busy and the strike was very stressful." I was afraid Miss Givens might slug her.

"Very well," Miss Larkin said brightly as we reached the ward door. "Keep fighting the good fight."

"We will, and thank you," I replied, actually pushing Miss Larkin out into the corridor. I heard Miss Givens heading our way.

I quickly closed and locked the door. "Who was that?" Miss Givens said, standing beside me. Miss Larkin was motoring down the hall like someone escaping a fire.

"That was Miss Larkin," I said, making certain to stand between Miss Givens and the doorhandle.

"Got her out of here pretty quick, didn't you?" Miss Givens said,

STEPHEN B. SEAGER, M.D.

glancing over my shoulder. "Afraid I might do something rash?" she added.

I only smiled. "You're learning," Miss Givens said and walked away.

V

It took awhile to assess exactly how I felt about the strike and the time I'd spent on Ward Three. First, it took me a week to catch up on my sleep and get back to any kind of personal routine. Second, and most importantly, it took some time to sift through my feelings and decide what, if anything, I'd learned.

Now I put it together like this. I felt good about the experience, really good. Not in the sense that I'd done anything outstanding or noteworthy, but good in the sense that I'd learned things that could not have been experienced any other way. It was an experience that, had I not gone through it, I would be a lesser person and certainly a poorer physician.

Many authors of note have also been physicians. Historically, Arthur Conan Doyle and Somerset Maugham come to mind. More recently, my favorite is Lewis Thomas. In all Dr. Thomas's work a common theme emerges, that of the dualism in medicine, the split between doctor as technician—remover of the appendix, reader of X-ray film—and the doctor as healer, as friend, as confidant. When did we substitute magnetic scanners for the laying on of hands, anyway?

This is not a new problem nor, certainly, am I the first one to pose it. But my two weeks of living on Ward Three got me thinking about it.

The main issue, I believe, is: What makes people well? Why do they get better? Corollary to this, of course, is why in this age of modern miracles do so many people remain sick? I read once that two-thirds of people suffering from depression never get treatment. How can that be?

I've decided that doctors, myself included, are mainly to blame. Somewhere along the line we lost sight of the forest for the technological trees. We assumed that the correct drug for the identified symptom was enough. That accurate diagnosis, scientifically arrived at, would, logically, lead to precise treatment and cure. We were wrong.

I used to tell this joke to young ER physicians. If, after you've ordered all the lab work, taken all the X rays, considered the opinions of your consultants, you're still confused about a diagnosis, as a last resort, talk to the patient. I used to tell that joke. And I used to laugh at it.

Anton Mesmer, an eighteenth-century Austrian physician, is called the father of modern hypnosis. He believed the therapeutic benefit derived from the trance state was the result of animal magnetism, an invisible fluid that passed between the hypnotist and subject. He called the process "mesmerism." I'm not sure he wasn't right.

As much as anything, the quality of a doctor's relationship with his patients is the best predictor of eventual outcome. Certainly, some patients recover in spite of you and others wither regardless of your efforts. But in the main, like Mesmer said, if there are good juices flowing between people, recovery is well on the way.

What a revelation this was to me that a relationship in and of itself can be therapeutic. That talking and caring really do help. That touching and listening and understanding are important. Bottom line, I learned that caring cures. That machines are no substitute for your time. That to get results you have to give. All the medicine in the world would not have helped Mae Peterson more than the time we spent talking. She knew it and now I do, too.

Which gets us back to this dualism business. Imagine the suffering that would be relieved if doctors could somehow learn to combine the two sides, scanners and compassion. The prospects are mind-boggling.

Everything in psychiatry these days is anatomically and biologically oriented, which is exciting and good. Most mental disorders can now be pinned on predictable pathology in a given neuron system or molecular group. For some diseases the defective gene may even have been located. I wouldn't find it surprising, then, if at some not too distant future date, an empathy center is located somewhere deep in the brain. It will be a tiny group of cells that secrete a very specific substance, a curamine, if you will, and it will prove to be the answer to what makes people well. There will be one catch, however: The empathy center will only work if acted upon by animal magnetism.

THIRTEEN

TIME BOMB TICKING

I

IT WAS A NEW YEAR on Ward Three, and after my experience with the strike I had to admit I was looking at the place differently or, more specifically, I was looking at my patients differently. I tried to be more in tune with their day-to-day problems and more receptive to concerns generated by just being on the ward itself. I started asking fewer questions about voices and strange beliefs and more about their opinions of the food. I told them I knew it was a scary place at night. I asked if their room was clean enough and how the staff was treating them. And, regardless of how bizarre or confused their answer was, I sat and listened.

Maxwell Jones, an English psychiatrist, was right on the mark about how I was feeling those first few weeks in January. War produces as many mental casualties as physical ones. Following World War II, Jones was faced with the catastrophic psychological aftermath of England's fight with Germany. There were simply too many patients and not enough professional staff.

Dr. Jones's solution to this dilemma would help shape the course of mental health treatment for years to come. He created what came to be known as the "therapeutic community." Therapeutic community means that the environment is part of the treatment.

With so few "officially" trained doctors and nurses, Jones made everyone part of the staff: social workers, janitors, clerks, and finally the patients themselves. In his democratic view, class and rank distinctions were dropped. All decisions were mutually discussed and concensually agreed upon. He believed this approach fostered independent thinking and action on the part of patients, which, in mental health treatment, is really your ultimate goal.

And that's how I began to feel about Ward Three. That we were a true community, all striving for a common purpose. All pulling together. I had this feeling for a few weeks. Then it went away. When Ward Three turned into Madison Square Garden.

II

I met Kesha Turner one night in late January when I was on call. The police brought her in on an involuntary hold. She'd been picked up at a local donut shop for creating a disturbance, apparently over the correct amount of her change. That's the report I got, anyway. It all seemed a little tame to me. I sensed there had to be more.

"Suspect Kesha Turner was observed at the above location," the policeman had written on her hold papers in that universal Joe Friday style. "Suspect was partially clothed. The location, J and B Donuts, was noted to be in disarray. Sales clerk at location appeared to be bleeding from the nasal area. When confronted, suspect shouted, 'God did it! God did it!' "

I happened to run into the same cop later in the evening and asked him about Kesha Turner. Basically, the story went like this. Kesha had gone to the donut shop just after eleven. She was agitated, pacing like a caged lion. Somehow she managed to place an order and wait for it to be filled. When the clerk shorted her a nickel in change, however, Kesha exploded. She started screaming and throwing donuts. She ripped off her shirt. She punched the clerk in the face. When the cops arrived, J and B Donuts was in ruins.

I was still fresh from my revelatory two-week stay on Ward Three and was feeling pretty competent that night. Psychiatry, I'd decided, was definitely my cup of tea. I wanted to savor every drop. I was a sponge ready to soak up experience. I was determined to interview Kesha Turner before making any decisions. I was determined to get to the bottom of this.

"You want me to take her downstairs?" a security guard up in triage asked.

"No. I'd like to speak with her first," I said.

"You want me to come in there with you?" the guard asked. "She looks a little wild."

"I think I can handle it. But thanks for offering," I said and then followed Kesha into the small interview room, closing the door behind me.

At that exact moment I learned the therapeutic community concept doesn't apply in emergency psychiatric settings. Or, if it does, Kesha Turner had never heard of it. "I'm Doctor Seager," I said, motioning for Miss Turner to sit. "How can I help . . ." was as far as I got before she spun around and punched me flush in the face.

As blood began dripping on my shirt, I quickly pinched my nose and scrambled from the room. The same security guard was just outside the door. He had a wad of Kleenex in his hand. "It usually takes one good bop before you learn," he said, handing me the tissues.

III

Kesha Turner suffered from borderline personality disorder. While not a true major mental illness like schizophrenia or bipolar disorder, it is, as the name implies, pretty close. "Borderlines," as they are called, spend a lot of time right on the edge.

The whole concept of personality disorders is interesting. These people suffer from one basic flaw in their psychological make up, their character. They tend to react to stress in the same predictable, dysfunctional way every time. They don't have the flexible array of responses that "normal" people do. They have, to be literary for a moment, that one "fatal flaw," a Hamlet kind of thing.

Historically, there has always been a sense that certain people have a pathological bent. The Greeks recognized four temperaments—sanguine, phlegmatic, choleric, and melancholic. The modern DSM-III-R classification system contains three groups or "clusters." First is the "odd" or eccentric group. These are people who, without showing signs of psychosis, are persistently suspicious, bizarre, or reclusive. They make good night watchmen or hermits.

The second group are pathologic extroverts. Borderlines fit into this category. These people are overly concerned with themselves. They lack conscience and empathy. They're egotistical. They can be irritatingly manipulative, dramatic, and flamboyant. They are, as a rule, fairly unstable. They are also, as a rule, real pains in the neck.

The last cluster is the ultimate introverts. They're avoidant, dependent, and overly passive. They are the quiet mice we tend to ignore, true flowers on the wall of humanity.

Freud said mental health was the ability to love and work. People with personality disorders generally have trouble in both areas. As a group they are a persistently annoying lot. They just can't get along with anyone.

Among personality disorders, borderlines are particularly malignant. They only feel comfortable when things around them are in turmoil. They are consumed by rage. They are impulsive. They are self-destructive. Drug use, reckless driving, suicide threats, and self-mutilation are their hallmarks. They feel chronically empty and bored. As one might guess, they have trouble maintaining stable relationships. They also, as Kesha Turner had done, occasionally cross the line into psychosis. Keeping borderlines on a locked ward is like trying to keep a cyclone in a bottle.

IV

I was having lunch in the main hospital cafeteria with Glen Charles and Dr. Ashwin when the announcement came over the common intercom. "Doctor Blue, Ward Three, Psychiatry. Doctor Blue, Ward Three, Psychiatry." Dr. Blue was the special code for anything requiring the immediate attention of hospital security. It generally meant a fight.

All three of us said the same thing as we stood from the table and ran. "Kesha Turner."

Kesha had been on the ward nearly a week. I'd put her on Haldol for her psychotic symptoms, and Klonopin, a long-acting Valium, to try and quiet her down. The Haldol was working fine, and all her talk about God had pretty well cleared up. But the Klonopin hadn't touched her. She'd stayed revved up from the moment she hit the ward.

Dashing across the street and into the psych building we were passed by a group of five security men, their short billy clubs at the ready. We took the stairs instead of the elevator. When we got to the ward it was all over but the shouting. Literally.

The hallway was full of panting guards and startled patients. The staff had locked themselves in the nursing station, except Miss Givens, who, as usual, had been right out in the thick of things.

"Kesha?" I said, picking Miss Givens out of the crowd.

"Who else?" Miss Givens muttered. She was still out of breath.

"How many days have we had to put her down in restraints?" I asked.

"How many days has she been here?" Miss Givens asked back. "Six."

"Then it's been six days."

Miss Givens had a look in her eye much like the one she'd given me that first morning in July. I read it as, "A real doctor wouldn't have let things get out of hand like this."

"Maybe I should do something about her medications," I said feebly.

Miss Givens didn't reply, but I sensed I'd hit the right area.

"Who'd she tangle with this time?" I finally asked.

Miss Givens had gotten her wind back. "Les O'Connor," she said as the security people began to leave. "She's working her way down the roster."

Kesha Turner had managed to alienate just about every patient and staff member on the ward. Each day, it seemed, she'd pick out a new target and, eventually, a brawl would result.

I wasn't surprised that Kesha had chosen to mix it up with Les O'Connor. Les, a rugged, hulking, red-headed Irishman, was a Vietnam vet who just couldn't shake the tortures of the war. He'd been in and out of County General for years. He had something of a short fuse. That he and Kesha Turner would square off was inevitable.

Judging from the looks of the dayroom, it must have been quite a battle. As I said, Les O'Connor was a big man and Kesha Turner was no skinny minny. Standing in the doorway I got a sense for what J and B Donuts must have looked like.

The chairs were scrambled around like eggs. One big table was overturned. Books and game pieces were everywhere. Now I knew why the ward TV was on a shelf high up on the wall. Had it been handy, either Turner or O'Connor would have been wearing it.

"Anyone hurt?" I asked Miss Givens who'd followed me in.

"The usual," she said, sadly surveying the mess. "Lots of damage, not much pain."

I'd noticed that when patients on the ward got violent they tended to vent their rage on the furnishings rather than each other. I knew, however, that I had to get Kesha Turner calmed down quick. She hadn't picked on Ricky Myers yet.

Both Les O'Connor and Kesha Turner had to be placed in four-point restraints and sedated. It took awhile, however, for the medication to work. So for the next twenty minutes we had to listen to our two combatants scream at each other.

"You stupid honkey bastard!" Kesha would bellow. "I'll stomp your ugly white rear end!"

"Try anything again, bitch," O'Connor would scream back, "and you'll be wearing my boot up your asshole."

And so on and so on. Finally the medicine kicked in.

V

I learned a great deal from Kesha Turner—some about her illness but mostly about myself. I learned why psychiatry takes years to master and why an understanding of your own quirks and problems is so important.

Kesha Turner really put me through my paces. I endured a period of feeling like a real sap, then came a time when I thought I was doing a truly fine job, and finally she made me feel like a jerk again. I nearly came to blows with Miss Givens while Kesha Turner was on the ward. The woman turned me inside out and back again.

As things on Ward Three generally did, it all began innocently enough. Two days after her row with Les O'Connor, after I'd stopped her Haldol and doubled the dose of Klonopin, Kesha was finally under control. At least I felt comfortable enough to sit across the desk from her in my office. I did, however, leave the door open.

"Did I do that?" Kesha said, pointing to the last remnants of black and blue around the bridge of my nose. I nodded my head.

"I'm awfully sorry," she said apparently sincerely. "Can you forgive me?"

For a moment I thought I was talking to the wrong person. During the past week I hadn't heard a civil word come out of Kesha Turner's mouth. Now she was being downright pleasant.

"It's alright," I said finally. "I don't think you knew what you were doing."

"I'm glad you feel that way," Kesha said. "I'd hate to lose you as my doctor. You're the best I've ever had."

Now I was really confused. All I'd done was load her up with medication and write for restraint orders. Since the night she'd tagged me, I couldn't remember a single sentence passing between us when she hadn't been strapped to the corners of her bed.

"I haven't done any . . ." I said before Kesha interrupted.

"Don't be so modest," she said sweetly. "All the patients say you're the best doctor up here. They always tell me how lucky I am." She was almost being coy.

And I bought her act hook, line, and sinker. "That's very flattering," I replied. I was getting some of that therapeutic community feeling back. "I do my best."

144

For the next hour our conversation went on exactly like that. Kesha Turner was charming, intelligent, and complimentary to a fault. I couldn't remember when I'd spent a more pleasant session with a patient.

Just as we were preparing to break, however, Kesha asked if I might do her a small favor. "Could you speak to Miss Givens, please," she said with a smile. "I'd like permission to go out on the patio during smoking break. Those cigarettes are killing me."

"Sure," I said. It seemed simple enough.

I brought up Kesha's request at the end of rounds the next morning. "I think we've finally turned the corner with Kesha Turner," I said proudly. "We spent a very productive hour yesterday in my office. She did have one request, however." I should have stopped at this point but didn't. I wasn't sharp enough yet to read body language. I didn't see Miss Givens's shoulders suddenly tighten, so I blithely pressed on. "She says during smoking times, the other patients' cigarettes really bother her. She asked if she might be taken to the patio. Would that be possible?" I asked.

Miss Givens didn't answer for a moment. I know now she was trying to keep from jumping up and strangling me. "No, that would not be possible," she said slowly. "I don't have the staff or the time to waltz Miss Turner outside because smoke bothers her. Besides," she added, "it's not ward policy."

Never being much of a stickler for policy and regulations myself, I thought Miss Givens was just being a little rigid. "I'm certain," I said with a tinge of irritation, "there's a way we can work this out."

This time Miss Givens was openly hostile. "No, Doctor Seager," was all she said.

This was definitely something new. For an instant, Miss Givens and I stared at one another, eye to eye. Maxwell Jones vs. Rules and Regulations. I felt a flush of anger rise in me. I'm certain Miss Givens was feeling the same thing. Fortunately, Dr. Ashwin defused the situation. "I'll talk to you after rounds," she said to me quietly and the tension subsided.

"Borderlines are splitters," Dr. Ashwin said as we sat in her office. There were ferns everywhere. "Do you know what splitting means?"

I had to confess I didn't. "Splitters thrive on disruption," she continued. "They split everything into either all good or all bad. And then they play both sides against one another."

"And right now I'm the all-good one," I said, remembering back to Kesha's flattering comments of the day before.

"Correct," Dr. Ashwin said softly. "And Miss Givens is the bad side. Kesha Turner is very bright," she went on. "She knows exactly the right buttons to push. Smoking really isn't the issue here. She was just testing the confrontational waters and," she said, looking at me directly, "if this morning is any indication, she may be onto something."

I felt awful. I hated myself for falling into Kesha's trap so easily, for being so gullible. But that didn't explain how I was feeling completely. I was feeling a little naked. I was upset that Dr. Ashwin and Kesha Turner could read me so easily. How would I ever become a psychiatrist if I were so psychologically porous?

Dr. Ashwin, as always, was quick to my rescue. "Don't worry," she said. "We've all fallen for this stuff ourselves. It's painful, I know. That's why we can see it happening in others."

I relaxed visibly. Dr. Ashwin had that effect on me. "I must warn you, however," she added in conclusion. "Borderline splitting goes both ways. Before this thing is over, you and Miss Givens will flip-flop roles. If Kesha senses that she's getting nowhere with you as the good doctor, you'll become the bad doctor real quick. Don't worry," she added with a smile. "You'll handle it."

For once Dr. Ashwin was wrong. I don't mean in the sense that her analysis and predictions weren't right on the mark, because they were. Events unfolded exactly like she said they would. I mean she was wrong when she said, "Don't worry. You'll handle it." At least I think she was wrong. She was wrong if her statement implied, "Don't worry. You'll handle it well."

FOURTEEN

STRANGE BEDFELLOWS

I

I FELT AN INSTANT kinship with Les O'Connor. He suffered from post-traumatic stress disorder or PTSD as it's come to be called. PTSD is not new. During WW I it was "shell shock." Following WW II, "combat fatigue." Only after adjustment problems experienced by Vietnam vets became so prevalent, however, was the issue ever studied in detail.

From all the recent books and movies about Vietnam, most people have some kind of feel for PTSD. PTSD implies that someone has been subjected to a severe stress, perhaps life-threatening, that goes beyond anything most people would ever encounter. Generally, this means war or natural disaster, but other things can certainly be included.

The psychic insult from such calamities can be so great that for months or years afterward these poor souls are wracked by flashbacks of sound, sight, smell, and emotion. They develop exaggerated, startle reactions. They avoid situations that might trigger a memory. They tend not to eat or sleep well. They are prone to severe depression.

Untreated, PTSD can be a seriously disabling illness. I know. I had a touch of it once myself.

I would never claim that nine years in the ER compares to actually facing combat—after all, my life was never on the line. But lots of other peoples' were. Day in and day out. Week after week. Month after month. Year after year. Continually balancing life and death may not equal facing a brigade of NVA regulars, but on the bell curve of severe stress, it's in there somewhere. At least it was for me.

The life of an ER doctor runs a predictable course. It's like the marathon. Eventually, somewhere along the line, you hit the wall. Generally, young, energetic doctors are attracted to the field; doctors who can't tolerate the confines of office or hospital practice. It's a real hands-on specialty. Things happen. Things move. It is, in the training experience of most medical students, the first place you feel somewhat competent, the first time you feel you're actually doing some good. For the uninitiated, ER medicine has a strong pull.

As time goes on, however, you see the flip side of the coin. Action means quick decisions. And decisions mean you'll eventually be wrong. Then, if you stay long enough, you'll be wrong again. And wrong again. It's just the mathematics of the situation. You can't fight it.

Soon this starts to prey on you. *I've been wrong before,* you say. *What if I'm wrong now? This is a crucial moment.* If you can't get past it, you're a goner. Personally, I think it's an enigma, incapable of solution. That's why you see so few old ER doctors.

The kids are first and always the worst. It's the way a family fixes their eyes on you the instant you step into that small, quiet, special waiting room. Telling a young couple their child is dead takes its toll. It's something you never get used to. The fiftieth time is no easier than the first. When the elderly died I found it particularly painful, too. After all, every patient is someone's mother, father, brother, or sister.

I knew it was over for me when an old gentleman passed away early one July evening. He'd become short of breath at home. His wife of fifty years dialed 911. Paramedics came and brought him to me. We did all we could; the man just died.

When I went to inform his wife, however, that's when I knew. She looked at me with such terror. "Am I actually going to hear those dreaded words?" her eyes said. And something in my mind simply said "No." Enough of this was enough.

I opened my mouth but nothing came out. Tears filled my eyes. My heart was suddenly racing. I thought I was going to faint. Maybe I did faint. I don't know. The next thing I remember was being back in the small call room sitting on the edge of the bed crying like a baby.

Somehow I collected myself and finished the shift. I phoned the hospital from home that night and said I wouldn't be in for work the next morning. Or ever.

I should have seen it coming but, I suppose, that's easy to say now. The bad dreams were first. Every night I woke up sweating. Then I developed a tic in my neck. My hands shook. I became frightened of the telephone. The sight of a hospital or the sound of an ambulance made me hyperventilate.

So when Les O'Connor spoke of his dreams and the intrusive, horrible images he experienced, I could relate. When he explained his phobias, I understood. We became close. We knew what each other was feeling.

Except in one area. We definitely had different taste in women. A few days after their big fight, Les O'Connor took up with Kesha Turner.

Sex is an issue infrequently discussed on a mental ward, but, like the atmosphere, it's always there. After all, the places aren't segregated by gender, and the patients are all locked in together, sometimes for months. It's inevitable that relationships form. And with relationships comes sex.

The subject of sex among patients is rarely discussed because it makes the staff so uncomfortable. The relationship of staff to patient on the ward is really a parent-child type thing. Patients are told when to eat, when to sleep, how to dress, what medicines to take, etc. And the staff gets comfortable with this. When sex is interjected, however, the delicate balance is seriously disrupted. It's like coming home and finding your daughter in bed with her boyfriend.

It wouldn't have been so bad, I suppose, if they just hadn't been so blatant about it. But Kesha Turner and Les O'Connor left no doubt about what was happening. They held hands. They necked openly in the courtyard. And we were forever running him out of her room at night. It all made for lively discussions during rounds.

"My nurses are really getting upset about Kesha Turner and Les O'Connor," Miss Givens said, I thought, to the general group gathered around the conference table. Then I noticed she was staring at me. I was startled. I hadn't really been paying attention.

"What?" I said, sitting up straight. Everyone was looking at me.

"What do you plan to do about Kesha Turner and Les O'Connor?" she repeated. "They're acting like two cats in heat."

Now I was really sweating. And I was a little upset, too. I thought this was something Miss Givens and I could have discussed in private. "What would you like me to do?" I asked.

"I'd like you to put an end to it," Miss Givens said sternly. "The other patients are all stirred up and they're driving the staff crazy."

Glen Charles looked a bit bemused. "I guess you'll have to move back onto the ward, Steve," he said with a smile. "To keep an eye on that girl." Everyone chuckled except Miss Givens.

"You're as much to blame as he is," Miss Givens said, her tone now more angry than firm. "That O'Connor man is yours. Can't you set him some limits?" She had that what-kind-of-a-doctor-are-you-anyway look on her face. It was not a look to which Dr. Charles took kindly.

" 'That O'Connor man,' 'limits,' " he said, staring directly back at Miss Givens. "These are two grown adults we're talking about here. What do I care if they have sex? Sex is part of life, Miss Givens."

"Well it's not part of life on my ward," Miss Givens snapped.

Then Dr. Charles said something he probably shouldn't have. "Are we pushing a hot button here?" he said calmly, and Miss Givens's eyes lit like a firecracker. She whipped around like an uncoiled spring. I thought she was going to jump across the table. Fortunately, Dr. Singh stepped in.

"Let's everyone calm down," he said quietly.

Allowing a moment for her anger to wane, Miss Givens finally settled back into her chair.

"I'll talk to Mr. O'Connor," Dr. Charles said, "and Doctor Seager will speak with Kesha. We'll see what we can do."

"Thank you," Miss Givens said curtly. She didn't speak for the rest of the hour.

I did take Kesha Turner into my office and Dr. Charles spoke with Les O'Connor. I have no idea how their conversation went but I doubt it was as bad as mine.

II

"There's something we need to talk about," I said as Kesha took the seat across from me at my desk.

"If it's about me and Les, I don't want to discuss it," she said in that hostile, irritating tone I hadn't heard in awhile.

"I think we need to bring it up, anyway," I said, using my best reasonable voice. "Miss Givens says that . . ."

"I've got no problem with Miss Givens," Kesha said angrily. "It's you doctors that are the problem around here . . ."

"But . . ."

"I take your medicines," Kesha continued. Now she was really wound up. "I sit in here and listen to your bullshit day after day. I eat your crappy hospital food. I do everything you and those two other fools tell me to do. But my personal life is my own business and I'll thank you to keep your nose out of it."

Now I was a little steamed, too. "Listen, Kesha," I said, "this is a hospital and hospitals have rules just like anywhere else. We may not like them but we all have to follow them. And sex between patients is one thing that's just not allowed."

"Patients!" Kesha said indignantly. "Is that all we are to you? Just a bunch of 'patients'? Let me tell you, Mr. High and Mighty Doctor Seager. We're people here, not patients. You go home every night to your cute wife and your cute kids in your cute house, but we don't. What do you know about being a patient here, anyway?"

"I know more than you think," I snapped. Kesha had sucked me in again and we were really going at it.

"I'll bet you do," she said snidely. "You get your horns clipped every night but you can't stand the thought of me, a patient, doing the same thing." Kesha put special emphasis on the word "patient."

"My life is not the issue here," I said. I'm certain you could hear my voice halfway down the hall. "You and Les O'Connor having sex here on Ward Three is. It's against the rules and it is going to stop, understand?"

Kesha looked me up and down for a moment. My face was flushed, my fists clenched. She'd won and knew it.

"Yes, Doctor Seager, I understand," she said melodramatically. Then she stood to leave. "I feel sorry for your wife," she added, going out the door. "You must be some lousy lay."

After Kesha was gone I looked myself up and down. Then I touched the sweat on my forehead. I took a couple of deep breaths and put my head on the desk. I didn't understand anything.

III

There is a difference between therapy and counseling. It's the reason most people think psychiatrists are evasive, always answering a question with a question. That, in fact, is what they're supposed to do.

Counselors give advice. Unsure about what to do? They'll tell you. This is comforting. This is helpful. This, however, is not therapy.

Therapy is giving a patient, through open-ended questions and carefully timed interpretations, the ability to solve their own problems. Its goal is emotional release, insight, and growth. I got a window into this process from my supervisor, Dr. Jefferson. I called his office right after my fiasco with Kesha Turner.

Dr. Jefferson smiled and leaned back, twining his fingers across his vest buttons as I sat in the upholstered chair beside his large mahogany desk. I smiled back.

"I'm having real trouble with one of my patients," I said when it became apparent that Dr. Jefferson wasn't going to speak first.

"I see," Dr. Jefferson said.

I felt a strong twinge of anxiety. "That's not really true," I said. "I'm having trouble with my reaction to one of my patients. She's a borderline and she's making me crazy. I don't like the way I feel about her."

Dr. Jefferson, a stately, bald black man in his mid-fifties, nodded. "How do you feel about her?" he asked.

I paused for a moment. "I hate her," I said finally, and was stunned by my answer. Doctors weren't supposed to hate patients. "I don't hate her," I fumbled. "I mean I'm not supposed to hate her but I guess I do." I felt some of the anxiety lessen.

"What do you mean by 'hate'?" Dr. Jefferson said.

"I mean she makes me angry and frustrated," I replied. The words were coming a little easier now. "She's unpredictable, manipulative, loud, and abrasive. I can't relate to her. I can't understand her so I can't help her. I don't know if I want to help her." I smiled a nervous smile. "I need your advice. Things are out of control."

"Is control an important issue with you?" Dr. Jefferson asked.

I thought for the longest time. "I guess it is," I said. "I imagine it is for everyone. Everybody likes to feel in control, to feel competent."

As that last sentence rolled out, it was like a buzzer suddenly went off in my head. "Control isn't really the issue, is it?" I said. It was a true moment of insight. "The issue is competence. She makes me feel insecure. Like I don't know what I'm doing. That's what I hate."

"And what are you doing with these feelings?" Dr. Jefferson asked. "Where do they go?"

This one was easy. "I heap them back on Kesha Turner," I said quietly. "She makes me feel insecure and I pay her back by hating her." It was like someone had switched on the lights.

"Does that answer feel good to you?" Dr. Jefferson asked.

The tension was completely gone. I really did feel good. "Yes, sir," I said. "Yes, it does."

"Then it's probably correct," Dr. Jefferson concluded.

And that's basically how the remainder of the hour went. I discussed some of my other patients and verbalized my feelings about them. I told him how I felt about being an intern, about working for the county, and about working at County General in particular. I told Dr. Jefferson how proud I was of the work Dr. Charles and I'd done during the strike and how close I'd felt to my patients during that time.

I explained my ambivalent feelings toward my budding relationship with Ricky Myers. Basically I got a whole load of stuff off my chest and all the while Dr. Jefferson never unlaced his fingers once.

I left my supervision session feeling much better. I was much clearer on how I felt. I had a good idea about how to proceed. And, best of all, I'd concluded that I was right where I was supposed to be in my training. That things were progressing down the correct path. I felt that, all in all, I was doing okay.

I was prepared to apply my new-found knowledge into forging a stronger and, hopefully, more therapeutic relationship with Kesha Turner. I was determined to do things differently from now on. But, as usual, Kesha beat me to the punch.

IV

I wasn't panicked by the blood. I'd worked ER long enough to know that when it's splattered on the floor, a little goes a long way. Miss Givens didn't seem all that upset, either. I think she was mainly concerned about the mess. But when Kesha Turner sliced her wrist in the dayroom that afternoon, it sure riled everyone else up.

People were yelling and hopping, frantically trying to get away or trying to help, all, it seemed, at the same time. The one truly calm person was Kesha Turner. With that small piece of metal in one hand and blood dripping from the other, she was cool as a cucumber. She looked relieved. Almost serene.

I saw Kesha just after she'd gotten back from the ER. There were thirteen fresh stitches beneath the white tape and gauze dressing around her wrist. She had a look of anticipation on her face as I walked into the room. I didn't know how she expected me to react, but for once, I think, she was wrong.

"That must be painful," I said, leaning on Kesha's nightstand and pointing to her wrist. She was sitting on the side of the bed.

"It's all your fault, you know," Kesha snapped. "You and the rest of this pissant staff around here."

"I'm sure you see it that way, Kesha," I said. "And you may be right." I quickly shifted to another subject. "You must have really been hurting to do something like that," I said sincerely.

Kesha Turner looked honestly surprised. She'd laid the trap and I hadn't fallen in. "I was angry at you and the staff," she said with rising emotion. "I was angry at everybody."

"So you took it out on yourself?" I asked.

With that, Kesha Turner broke down and wept. I didn't feel manipulated. I didn't feel angry. For the first time since I'd known her, I felt sorry for Kesha. And for the first time since I'd known her I got an honest glimpse at the terror she must have felt.

Things went better for Kesha and me after that. She didn't change much but I did. I apologized to Miss Givens, then as a unit, the staff sat down and mapped out a common strategy for managing Kesha. We finally had a united front.

We set limits and stuck by them. There were no favors granted, no sides taken. Problems were discussed the moment they came up. We didn't allow even the smallest wedge to be driven between us.

Oddly, during the remainder of her stay on the ward, Kesha kept up her romance with Les O'Connor. You never saw the two apart. They were the real "Odd Couple."

When Kesha was finally discharged, Les O'Connor, a voluntary patient, signed himself out the same day.

I mentioned that borderlines have trouble with relationships. They can start them alright; it's maintenance that's the problem. I ran into Les O'Connor at a local market some time later. "You still seeing Kesha Turner?" I asked.

"Are you kidding?" O'Connor said with a pained laugh. "That woman's crazy."

FIFTEEN

KRYPTONITE

I

AFTER WORKING WITH Glen Charles for two months I could honestly say that he lived up to his advance billing. The man was brilliant. At rounds, he and Dr. Singh's thorough dissection of each case—psychodynamics, genetics, social issues, medications—were simply inspiring. Unconsciously, I suppose, I began to see Glen as a role model. I can't remember ever being more impressed with a man. That's why the fault lay as much with me as with him. Dr. Charles's light was so bright it blinded me.

I was fortunate enough to be present at Dr. Charles and our department's shining hour. It came one day in early February. As a senior resident he was often called in to consult on the various medical and surgical services across the street. There were other senior residents, of course, but word travels fast at The Bin and generally the requests came to Glen by name. And as his ward intern I got to go along.

Our consultation work was fascinating. The reasons other doctors call in a psychiatrist are many and varied but, after a while, I did notice one common theme. Generally, the psychiatrist is called upon to fill in for defects in the other doctor's personality.

I hate to keep harping on the importance of the doctor-patient relationship, that animal magnetism stuff, but it's just so important. And never was the miserable state of this crucial element so glaring as when I followed Dr. Charles on his consultation work.

We were asked to inform patients that they had cancer and were going to die. We were expected to tell people they were about to lose a limb or needed surgery. All the bad news that these poor doctors couldn't handle themselves. What does it say, I began to wonder, about a surgeon's rapport with his patient when he must bring in a total stranger to discuss diagnosis and treatment?

Another point became readily apparent as well. Some other doctors, especially the older ones, really don't think much of psychiatrists. And, to a degree, this is understandable, I suppose. In the past, before the recent explosion in the neurosciences, psychiatry was really the stepchild of medicine. Why would anyone (a "real" doctor is the intended meaning) suffer through medical school just to spend their day chatting? Psychiatry, so went the assumption, was the repository of those who couldn't cut it anywhere else.

Things, of course, are vastly different now. Freud's couch has been replaced by scanners and receptor assays. A good modern psychiatrist knows as much about the patient as a whole, including all his physical maladies, as anyone. This point was hammered home one afternoon when Dr. Charles was asked to see a man in the surgical ICU. The consultation request was marked "Urgent."

Of all the doctors who're weird about psychiatrists, surgeons top the list. It's like oil and water. The ultimate talkers vs. the ultimate doers. They won't say it, but I suspect they think we're wimps. This particular case was no different. The patient, Juan Gonzalez, had been admitted for stomach pains and vomiting. During the course of his workup, however, Mr. Gonzalez had taken a turn for the worse. He was suddenly delirious and was running a high fever. His muscles were getting rigid. A CAT scan of his abdomen revealed nothing. When his blood pressure began to fluctuate, things got very tense. In desperation, exploratory surgery was planned. Juan Gonzalez was fifty-four and if something wasn't done quickly, he wasn't going to see fifty-five.

This impending surgery was how we got involved with the case. The surgeons wanted us to explain things to an hysterical family. Dr. Weber, chief surgical resident, asked us to specifically mention that Mr. Gonzalez might die.

With a smile, Dr. Charles said we'd be happy to do what they asked. Maintaining good relations with the other hospital departments was paramount at County General. Doctors were reluctant enough to come onto the psych wards when we needed them. Bad feelings would only make matters worse. So Glen Charles explained the situation to the Gonzalez family. Then we rejoined the surgeons in the ICU. They were at the bedside.

"Mind if I look at the chart?" Dr. Charles said and the surgical intern gave him a funny look.

"Think this is the result of some deep-seated neurotic conflict?" Dr. Weber said with a laugh.

Glen Charles smiled back. "You never know," he said, picking the chart off the bed and flipping a few pages.

Soon the surgical team was engrossed in a discussion about abdominal pathology, occasionally pointing to or poking at Mr. Gonzalez like he was a demonstration dummy. All the while Dr. Charles was studying the chart.

"How long has he been getting Compazine?" Glen said finally, looking up from Mr. Gonzalez's medication sheet.

"What?" Dr. Weber said. He seemed a bit annoyed that we were still hanging around. I think he wanted to say, "You've done your job, now toddle off."

"How long has Mr. Gonzalez been getting Compazine?" Glen persisted.

"Mr. Gonzalez has been on Compazine for a week. Why?" Weber said. He was obviously irritated.

"I think your patient has NMS," Dr. Charles said.

"What's NMS?" Weber asked disdainfully.

"Neuroleptic Malignant Syndrome," Glen replied calmly. Until recently, NMS was only mentioned in the fine print of textbooks. "NMS is a rare, unexplained bad reaction to neuroleptic medication," Dr. Charles explained. "Compazine is a neuroleptic, like Thorazine. High fever, delirium, muscle rigidity, vital-sign instability, it all fits."

At this Dr. Weber became almost hostile. "Thanks for the input, Doctor Charles," he said, leaning down to read Glen's name tag. "Now, if you'll excuse us please, we have work to do."

For just an instant I saw some of the old football player in Glen Charles's eyes. "After you open him up and find nothing," Glen said, carefully placing the chart back on the bed, "and before Mr. Gonzalez dies, you call me again and we'll discuss NMS."

"Surgeons are swine," Dr. Charles said on the way back to Ward Three. He checked his watch. "It's eleven now," he said. "Give them two hours for surgery. Two hours to pick their noses. They'll phone back by four."

Actually we got the call at four-thirty. And this time there was an entirely different feel to the group that gathered around Mr. Gonzalez's bed.

Dr. Weber was there, his smug look having turned to mild pallor. His "boss," Dr. Horowitz, a short, pudgy man of fifty, was there. Three junior residents were there also, all in a row.

These guys were obviously sweating bullets.

Glen Charles showed real class. He could have rubbed it in good but he didn't. He just got down to business.

"NMS is a reaction to the dopamine receptor blockade properties of neuroleptic medications," he began. "What was overlooked here is the fact that the Compazine you used to treat this man's nausea is really a neuroleptic." Well, he got in a little dig.

For the next fifteen minutes Dr. Charles gave a dissertation on the cause, diagnosis, treatment, and management principles of NMS. He gave detailed descriptions for the use of dantrolene, a muscle relaxer, and bromocriptine, a dopamine helper, the two drugs used in combination being the best method of attack. He tied everything up nicely at the end. "If it's not too late already, I think we've got a good chance to save Mr. Gonzalez." I guess a second dig was understandable.

Dr. Horowitz thanked Dr. Charles as did Dr. Weber, albeit somewhat grudgingly. He knew what was in the offing, and as Glen and I walked down the hall we discovered why the chief surgical resident had been so uneasy.

We listened to Dr. Horowitz's tirade all the way to the elevators. We didn't catch everything but we got the highlights. "A goddamned psychiatrist!" he kept shouting over and over.

II

Mr. Gonzalez did fine after that. He slowly turned the corner and came out of his funk. We visited every morning—somehow, it seemed, always when Dr. Weber wasn't around. In a week, Mr. Gonzalez was up and talking. "I don't need a psychiatrist," he said when Dr. Charles and I walked into the room one morning. "I'm not crazy."

"We're here if you need us," Dr. Charles said politely and we excused ourselves. "I wonder if he'll ever know what really happened?" I asked as we left the surgical floor.

Dr. Charles only smiled. It was a stupid question.

What's ironic is that it happened that very same day. The day of such success with Mr. Gonzalez. It almost makes you think there's a ledger somewhere. That someone likes to keep the books balanced.

Millie Jensen was an average-sized black woman with skin the color of polished ebony. She was forty but looked fifty. She'd come from a prominent Atlanta family. Someone said her father had been a judge.

Like Mae Peterson, Millie Jensen was a victim of the drift down theory. Also, like Mae Peterson, recurrent bouts of severe depression had been her ticket on the Big Bin Express.

Millie was a patient of Dr. Charles's. I never really got to know her well. I did, however, follow her progress from reports at rounds and, of course, that one day I glanced at her chart.

Anti-depressant medications work. How they work is another story. Within a month, seventy percent of the most severely depressed people generally respond. They are, in my book, true wonder drugs.

They are also very complicated drugs. Their pharmacokinetics are tricky, their side effects can be serious. They're not for use by the uninitiated. Glen Charles knew them backwards and forwards. Over the past two months, I'd heard him discuss each of the dozen or so medications in minute detail. I'd paid special attention to his caveat about one problem most of the drugs had in common. If he'd said it once he'd said it a thousand times. "Anti-depressants are cardio-toxic," i.e., in high doses they are poison to the heart. They delay the organ's electrical conduction system. This can lead to heart block. Which can lead to death.

Dr. Charles put Millie Jensen on nortriptyline, a good drug but one with two unusual properties. First, the normal dose is lower than most anti-depressants. Whereas other compounds reach maximal efficacy at 200–300 mg, nortriptyline requires only 150 mg, about half that. Second, the drug has what's called a "therapeutic window." This means you get your best response with blood levels in a narrow range. Below that range the drug won't work, nor, interestingly, will it work at levels above the window.

Such was my respect for Glen Charles that I didn't even believe what I saw. I knew my eyes, not Glen Charles's, had been wrong. Even when I discussed it with my wife that evening I wasn't sure.

"The man's not God," she said. "If he screwed up, you'd better tell somebody."

Even then I didn't call. I wanted to give my eyes one more check. This decision nearly cost a life. And not that of Millie Jensen.

"Oh, God," I moaned and actually let the chart slip from my hand. A dozen sheets of paper scattered across the floor. I'd come in early. Only Miss Givens and I were in the nursing station. "What's the matter?" she said, turning around from her desk.

"Has Millie Jensen had her morning dose of nortriptyline yet?" I asked. There was honest panic in my voice.

"Of course," Miss Givens said, looking at the wall clock. "You know that." She stood up. "Why?" she asked. "What's happened?"

I picked through the pile of papers around my feet until I found the green order sheet. "Read this," I said, handing it to Miss Givens.

"Oh, no," she said quietly.

There it was plain as day. Just like I'd seen it the day before but had refused to believe it. The order read, "Nortriptyline 150 mg BID," for twice a day. It should have read, "Nortriptyline 150 mg QD," for once a day. And the order was signed "Glen Charles, M.D." Millie Jensen had been getting twice the normal amount of medicine.

Instantly Miss Givens and I were tripping over each other to get to the phone. She called for a stat EKG. I phoned the lab to draw an immediate drug blood level, then I notified the ER that we had a patient on the way.

Finally we headed for Millie Jensen's room and both heaved an audible sigh of relief when we found her lying quietly in bed. After an apology by me for our screw-up, Miss Givens got Millie Jensen ready to travel.

Mercifully, X ray and lab arrived in no time and quickly finished their jobs. When Millie stood up to get into a wheelchair, however, she fainted back onto the bed. "Get a gurney," I shouted to a passing attendant. "And hurry." I looked at Millie's EKG. Things were bad. The current in her heart was barely moving.

"Get the crash cart ready," I said to Miss Givens as the rolling bed arrived. "We may have a cardiac arrest."

Fortunately, we didn't. Millie, two attendants, and Miss Givens got safely off and out the door. Two minutes later, Dr. Charles and Dr. Singh arrived on the ward. They came through the door together. Both were laughing.

Then Dr. Charles saw me standing in Millie Jensen's doorway with the emergency EKG in my hand. "What happened?" he said quietly.

III

Millie Jensen did fine. She was transferred to the medical ICU for a couple of days, where they continuously monitored her heart rate and blood pressure. Initially, there was talk of a pacemaker but one was never needed. The crisis gradually passed and she came back to Ward Three.

To his credit, Glen Charles seemed to do pretty well, too. These kinds of mistakes, the ones where a patient's life is threatened, can sometimes have a strange effect on doctors. A few never regain their confidence. But Glen Charles was Glen Charles. I wouldn't have expected any less.

Dr. Charles assumed full responsibility for the problem even after Miss Givens and I both apologized profusely for not picking it up sooner. He explained things in detail to Millie Jensen who said she understood. Dr. Singh put a cap on the whole affair during rounds. "Fortunately, nothing disastrous happened," he said. "Everybody makes mistakes. We're all only human." And that, it seemed, was the end of it.

One of the resident's duties on night call was to see consultation requests in the main hospital ER, a task I tried scrupulously to avoid. There were just too many bad memories. Too many ghosts. But every now and then the job fell to me.

Mainly, the ER wanted us to evaluate suicide attempts. We saw a lot of wrist cutters and pill takers—the most prevalent, nonfatal method of self-harm. They are commonly lumped under the term "suicide gestures," the implication being that these people only made a token effort, generally, it's assumed, to get somebody's attention. Troubled teenage girls do this frequently.

In psychiatry, however, you're taught to take every suicide attempt seriously, regardless of method. After all, if someone is willing to open up their wrist just to get attention, something is wrong somewhere. While all attempts may be equal, to paraphrase Orwell, some are more equal than others. If the threat or attempt involves a method that, once initiated, cannot be stopped—a gunshot, hanging, jumping off a building—these are taken very seriously.

Suicide is a particularly tragic psychiatric problem. In 1985, 28,500 Americans were known to have taken their own life. The number of attempts may be ten times that total. It's the eighth leading cause of death in this country. Like any other disease there are risk factors and different distribution patterns around the world.

Oddly, there is a "suicide belt," running from Scandinavia through Germany and into Eastern Europe. The incidence of suicide in these countries is twice that of the U.S. Men kill themselves more frequently than women, although women have many more attempts. The majority of suicides occur between ages fourteen and forty-four.

Rates among the young, especially urban blacks, and those over eighty are rapidly rising.

The nineteenth-century sociologist Emile Durkheim made the first major contribution to the study of suicide. He related the act to a person's alienation from society. Freud said it was anger toward another directed against self. Menninger called it "inverted homicide." Before you kill yourself, they say, you must have a repressed desire to kill someone else. And if events of the next few days were any indication, these theories were on the right track.

SIXTEEN

A HURRICANE BREWING

I

IT WASN'T THE actual patient I was called to see that night in the ER, or the wild incident that followed, or even the gun shots that stuck most in my mind the next morning. I'd come to expect the bizarre as normal at The Bin. What stayed with me the next day was something smaller, something seemingly innocuous. Something that could easily have been forgotten.

On my way to the ER I passed by medical records. The door was open. A light was on. I stuck my head inside. Glen Charles was sitting at a small table filled with charts he'd pulled from the canyons of files behind him. He smiled when he saw me. "Catching up on a little dictation," he said.

I checked the clock. It was nearly ten. "Go home and get some sleep," I said, smiling back. "See you in the morning."

What bothered me was that Dr. Charles was still in medical records when I came back an hour later. And the pile of charts in front of him had grown even larger. There was something about the look on his face that said he didn't want to be disturbed. So I left him alone. This was a mistake.

169

II

Just the sight of the main hospital ER made my skin crawl. First, it was the nervous crowd standing outside smoking and pacing. Waiting. Those people outside all had people inside. People at the end of IV lines, attached to beeping machines. It was a scene I'd seen a million times before.

I hesitated before crossing the street. It was suddenly all coming back to me. As I stared at that big red EMERGENCY sign, I began to breathe fast. My heart was really pumping. Then it all went away. It went away because I realized in that ER I wasn't the one in charge. I wouldn't have to speak to all those people waiting outside. I wouldn't be the one to give them the bad news. I was only going in to see one patient. They only wanted my advice. Then I could go. I quickly strode across the street and through those two big swinging doors.

Walking into the main ER on a Friday night was like walking into a Dali painting. The place is that surreal. I half expected Rod Serling to appear.

The best description I can conjure is that of a human beehive if you also throw in a dozen people shouting at once, women weeping and moaning in Spanish, a bank of phones ringing, gurneys thumping like bumper cars, IV bottles flying, blood dripping, X rays clicking. And all the while those doors just keep bringing in more.

Amid the din I managed to locate a harried ER resident. He looked like I used to feel. "I'm Doctor Seager from psychiatry," I said. "You have a patient for me to see?"

"Her chart's here somewhere," he said, shuffling through a stack of metal-covered files scattered in a heap on the nursing station counter. Then he took a quick phone call and returned to the search. "Here it is," he said at last. Then he looked at me and sighed. "Psych, huh?" he lamented. "That must be the life."

"Stop over after your shift," I said with a grin. "We're just firing up the hot tubs." I thought the ER guy would laugh, but he didn't. He just kept looking at me.

I found my patient, Talitha Harper, on a gurney pushed up against a far wall. Hers was one of a number of gurneys lining the walls, filling the corridors and stuffed into corners. Every regular bed had, of course, long since been filled. Talitha Harper was thirty-four years old. She'd cut her wrist with a razor blade. There were four identical scars beside her new stitches. Her forearm looked like a railroad track.

I noticed she had leather restraints on her legs. After introducing myself I inquired about them. "I don't know," she said quietly. "I guess they thought I was going to run."

I knew this was not an uncommon ER practice. With so many patients and so few staff, expedience is often the operative word. "Have you been depressed?" I asked.

And immediately tears came to the woman's eyes. Depression is peculiar. People rarely know they have it until someone asks. And once they do, the floodgates open.

I just let Talitha Harper talk. She told me one of those stories so common in the ghetto. She'd never known her father. High school dropout. Sexually abused as a child. Pregnant at seventeen. Five children before thirty. An alcoholic boyfriend who beat her. She was facing eviction. She slashed her wrist.

I truly sympathized with Talitha Harper and was impressed by her fortitude. Given her story, I'd have put a .45 in my mouth years ago. We were discussing admission plans when the ER doors suddenly burst open like they'd been set with dynamite.

Instantly everyone froze as three angry young black men stormed inside with four equally angry young cops right behind them. It was the Blues after a Red or the Reds after a Blue. Either way, we were in for big trouble.

The human instinct for survival, I knew, was a strong force. Until that night, however, I never realized just how powerful it could be. That's what makes bravery in the face of danger all that more remarkable. I guess that's why they give out combat medals.

I learned a great deal about courage in those next few moments. Basically, I learned I didn't have any. Nor, it seemed, did anyone else.

When the lead cop reached out and grabbed the last young man by the shoulder, everything exploded. Punches were flying, people were screaming, bodies were rolling on the floor. Chairs and gurneys crashed like cars in a high-speed freeway accident. The battle raged from one end of the ER to the other and back again.

At least I think that's what was happening. It sounded like it, anyway. I can't tell you for sure because I really didn't see any of it. After the initial blow was thrown, I dove into a small room full of plaster-cast supplies.

I had lots of company, too. Before the melee was over, there were three nurses, a secretary, two orderlies, and another doctor in there with me. At the first sign of trouble, the entire ER staff had abandoned ship.

Later we felt a little ashamed, of course, leaving all those patients to their own devices, and especially Talitha Harper who was strapped to her bed. But, at the time, we were feeling something entirely different. What we were feeling was terror. Everyone knew what happened when you mixed gangsters and cops.

And, as always, it happened. The three shots came in that familiar *pop-pop-pop* sequence. There was another burst of screams followed by total silence. My heart was a bass drum.

"We've got an injured man," someone finally shouted and he sounded like a cop. One of the ER people gingerly opened the cast room door, then dashed outside. I was the last one to leave.

I remember two things from the next few minutes. I remember how impressed I was at the organized, precise response of the trauma team. The young man who'd been shot was off the floor and into the trauma room in no time. Like a well-oiled machine, the ER crew began IVs, took X rays, and hung blood. Before I'd even caught my breath, it seemed, the injured man was on his way upstairs for surgery. It was obvious they'd had way too much practice with this sort of case.

The second thing I remember is Talitha Harper's eyes. They were wide and unblinking. Like the eyes desert jackrabbits get in your headlights just before you flatten them.

I looked in those eyes for the longest time. "Get me out of here," Talitha finally said.

I looked down at her bandaged wrist, thought back to the description she'd given of her life, gazed briefly around the mangled ER, then looked back into Talitha Harper's eyes. She wanted out of more than County General Hospital.

III

It was funny. I quickly came to realize that I knew a lot of things *about* Glen Charles but that I didn't *know* Glen Charles. And, as I came to find out, neither did anyone else. I knew he'd played football. I knew he was an Ivy League grad. I knew he was a great doctor. But I didn't know where he lived. Or if he had a girlfriend. That sort of thing. In the end, it turned out what I didn't know about the man was much more important than what I did.

It was the night I saw him in medical records that got me thinking. When I saw him there again the next night, I began to wonder. On the third night I definitely knew something was wrong. But what could I do? Everytime I asked, Glen gave me the same answer: "Dictation." I'd worked at The Bin long enough to know that no one had that much dictation.

It wasn't anything I could really put my finger on. There was nothing obviously wrong with the man. He was still sharp as a tack at rounds. He looked fine. And he continued to get along great with the staff and his patients. But I just had this sense. A tiny warning light kept flashing somewhere in the back of my mind. A little voice kept telling me to worry.

Finally, that little voice got so loud I couldn't ignore it any more. I started down toward medical records. Fortunately, I knew the clerk, Carla Martinez, fairly well.

"I've seen Doctor Charles down here a lot recently," I said. It was early on a Wednesday morning in late February.

Carla, a cute, young Hispanic woman, stopped working at her computer and looked up. "He's been here every night for a week," she said. "Is he doing some kind of research project?"

That was a possibility I'd overlooked. "Might be," I said, my hopes rising. "What kind of charts does he ask for?"

Carla suddenly looked worried. "Is this important?" she said, glancing quickly from side to side like they do in the movies. We both knew she wasn't supposed to give out that kind of information.

I thought for a minute. It was that little voice again. "Yes, it's very important," I said finally.

"He asked to see charts on all his patients," Carla said.

"You mean all the patients since he's been on Ward Three?" I said.

"No. All his patients," Carla persisted.

"All his patients from this year?" I said.

"All his patients."

"Since he came here four years ago?"

Carla nodded. "All his patients," she said quietly.

Now I really had a bad feeling.

IV

"I could get in big trouble for this, sir," Ben said after I'd apologized for waking him.

"It's really important, Ben," I said anxiously. "You know I wouldn't ask otherwise."

Ben stared at me for a moment, then reached into his small nightstand. "Is Doctor Charles in some kind of trouble?" he said, handing me the key to Glen's office.

"I hope not," I replied and headed back upstairs.

The strangest feeling came over me as I slid Ben's key into Dr. Charles's office door. Twice I put it in only to pull it out again. I wanted to know and then again I didn't. On the one hand, I knew Glen Charles was a grown man and could take care of himself. What business did I have, I thought, meddling in his affairs, let alone snooping through his office. On the other hand, there was that little voice. I put the key in the lock a third time and turned the handle.

It didn't take long to find it. There, amid the stacks of journals and textbooks on top of Glen's desk, was a blue spiral notebook, the kind we all used in high school. I took a breath and opened it.

It was truly an amazing feat, one driven either by compulsion or panic, I wasn't sure which. Filling that notebook, page after page, in Glen Charles's distinctive, precise handwriting, was the name, diagnosis, admission date, discharge day, and, most importantly, a listing of every medication ever given to any of his patients. The dose and patient reaction were noted as well. It was incredible.

I was all the more frightened when I flipped to the back and read the last entry. It was Millie Jensen's. Nortriptyline 150 mg BID was circled in red.

I was scared and confused. I knew the mistake with Millie Jensen's medication had obviously affected Glen Charles much more than he'd let on. There was something very bad bubbling beneath that smooth surface. But knowing that didn't help much. "Glen, I broke into your office last night and read the crazy notebook," wasn't going to do it. I didn't know what it was, but something had to be done. That little voice was screaming like a siren.

I spent a sleepless night. Once again it was my wife who gave me a level-headed answer. "It sounds like this guy could use a friend," she said the next morning. "Talk to him."

I waited until we were alone in the conference room after rounds.

"Glen," I said as Dr. Charles stood to leave. "Can I speak with you a moment?"

"Sure. What is it?" Glen said, sitting back down.

"I was wondering," I said, battling that "Dr. Charles" image as hard as I could, "if you might not want to talk."

"Talk?" Glen said a bit uneasily. "You mean about a patient?"

"In a way," I replied. "I thought you might want to talk about this Millie Jensen business."

Glen hesitated for a split second. For just an instant, something almost came out. But then the door slammed shut again. "I appreciate your asking," he said and seemed sincere. "It's something that happened. Luckily no one was hurt. I've made mistakes before, I'm sure I'll make them again." The tone of his voice changed ever so slightly when he said that last part.

"You sure?" I said, giving it one more go.

This time there was no hesitation. "Very sure," Glen said. Then he smiled and changed the subject. "You know, I'll be finished here in a couple of months," he said.

"I know," I replied. "Things will never be the same."

"Thanks," Glen said. "Anyway, I want to give you my set of Robbins and Dexter. It helped me when I was starting out. I thought you could get some use out of it. It's practically yours already," he added with a laugh. "You've borrowed it enough."

I was stunned. Robbins and Dexter was a three-volume text of psychiatry. It was the bible for our profession. It cost a small fortune. "I couldn't do that, Glen," I stammered. "Those books are too expensive. Besides . . ."

Glen cut me off. "I won't hear another word about it," he said firmly. "The books are yours. You've earned them. You're the best intern I've ever worked with."

I was flattered beyond description. That Dr. Charles image had me once again firmly in its grasp. "Thank you," I mumbled.

"It's settled then," Glen said, shaking my hand and smiling. He stood up. "Gotta go," he said. "Appointments to keep. Appointments to keep."

It was the little Robert Frost-like statement Glen Charles made just before leaving the conference room that finally turned things around. After deciding that perhaps my fears about Glen had been overblown, I finished the day in relative peace.

When I finally left the hospital I decided to drive by the beach before going home. It was something I'd been doing more and more of lately. It was a clear, convertible-top-down, mild California winter night, the kind that makes you think about L.A.'s good things. As I was slowly cruising past the sand and distant rippling water, I let my mind wander. Then the concluding lines of the poem hit me. Had Dr. Charles been complete, he would have said, "I've got appointments to keep. And miles to go before I sleep. And miles to go before I sleep."

I slammed on my brakes, spun around, and headed back toward County General.

V

I quickly realized the significance of our short conversation that morning. Glen Charles wasn't giving me his beloved set of texts. He was bequeathing them. As I skidded into the nearly empty parking lot, I was furious at myself for not pressing Glen harder, for not doing enough, not caring enough. I was angry that I'd let his image overwhelm me. And for the first time I realized what a miserable burden it must have been to constantly hold it up from the other side.

I raced into the hospital, up the stairs, onto the ward and into my office. Panting like a dog, I reached for the phone. Then in a moment of confusion I realized I didn't know who to call. I'd never spoken to Glen Charles outside the hospital and wasn't sure I knew anyone that had.

Operator information had no listing for a Glen Charles, M.D. I got Dr. Ashwin at home. She didn't have his number, either. But she caught the tension in my voice. "This is about Millie Jensen, isn't it?" she asked, and I said yes. "I had a hunch something wasn't right," she said sadly. "I just didn't think it was my place . . ."

"I know the feeling," I interrupted. There wasn't time for talk. Dr. Ashwin asked what she could do. I told her to call the other residents. Someone had to have Glen's phone number. She suggested I try Miss Givens. I told her I'd wait thirty minutes for her return call.

"Talk to the nursing supervisor," Miss Givens said without asking any questions. "She has all the doctors' numbers." I expected her to mention something about me disturbing her at night but she didn't. "Good luck," was all she said before hanging up.

There is a term in psychiatry called "concrete thinking." It comes from the work of Piaget, a French psychologist who studied the development of thinking and reasoning patterns in children. He labeled one phase the "concrete operational" stage. This, he said, is a time when children cannot reason abstractly, cannot see cause and effect, can only deal with the here and now.

Many adults seem to have regressed back to this period. We've all dealt with them. They fit nicely into the slots of a bureaucracy. I'd run

178

into a number of them at County General already, but none quite as bad as Harriet Greenwell, RN, the evening supervisor of nursing.

I got her on the line the minute I hung up from Miss Givens. Without going into detail I explained the urgency of my plight.

"I'm not authorized to give out doctors' personal numbers," Miss Greenwell said curtly. I felt my blood begin to boil.

"This may be life or death," I pleaded, hoping to find a spark of humanity in the woman. It was a futile plan.

"Without a 229 form from Doctor Charles authorizing release," Nurse Greenwell said, "there's nothing I can do. I'm sorry."

I was suddenly enraged. "Goddamn it!" I shouted. "You've got the number and I'm going to get it if I have to come down there and rip it out of your hands!"

Even threats wouldn't budge her. "If you come near my files," she said calmly, "I'll call security and have you arrested."

And I knew she wasn't kidding. I slammed the receiver down so hard, the phone nearly went crashing to the floor.

I checked my desk clock. I still had fifteen minutes to wait for Dr. Ashwin's call. I didn't know what to do with myself. I was bursting with anger and frustration. I paced back and forth across the room. I tried to sit down but it only got worse. Then it erupted. I smashed the closest wall with my fist.

Then the phone rang. "Sorry, no luck," Anita said.

"Thanks for trying." I sighed and slumped into a chair. My hand was killing me.

SEVENTEEN

GLEN FACES THE ABYSS

I

AFTER A WHILE, a strange sort of calm came over me. It was almost like a Zen state, a sensation of succumbing to the Fates, of realizing the die is cast and there's nothing you can do about it. It must be the sense behind the old newspaper phrase, "The condemned man ate a hearty meal."

What I really needed was someone to talk to. I could have called my wife or gotten Dr. Ashwin again. I might even have phoned Miss Givens. But I knew I needed someone different. I needed someone with a longer perspective. Someone who'd seen the big picture. Besides, I had the perfect excuse. I hadn't returned the key to Glen Charles's office from the night before.

"You look troubled, sir," Ben said, taking back the key and putting it on his ring.

I sat on Ben's bed. "I'm worried about Doctor Charles," I said sadly. "This business with Millie Jensen's medication really threw him. I don't think he's used to making mistakes."

Ben only nodded. "He's quite a man, old Glen," he said, and I agreed.

"I knew his father," Ben said matter-of-factly. "Years ago. Back before . . . you know."

I couldn't believe my ears. "You knew Glen Charles's father?" I said incredulously.

"Meanest son of a bitch that ever drew breath," Ben said, practically spitting out the words. "Broke down his wife. Drove those kids so hard, nearly broke them, too."

"Go on," I said. "Please."

"That boy could never please the man," Ben continued. "Nothing was ever good enough for Sam Charles. Not football. Not medical school. Not anything. Why do you think he came to work here at County General?" Ben asked. "The boy could have gone anywhere. Just to please that miserable SOB, that's why."

Now I was confused. "I thought you hadn't left the hospital in thirty years," I said. "How do you know all this?"

"Glen and I spent hours talking," Ben said.

"I've never seen you say more than hello and goodbye," I said. Then it all became clear. "He knows about you, doesn't he?" I asked.

"Yes, sir, he does," Ben replied. "I invited him down just after his father passed . . ."

"Glen's father is dead?" I asked, interrupting.

"Two years ago, sir," Ben said flatly. "Shot dead on the street. Poor Glen felt responsible. He'd always said when he became a doctor he'd move his family out of there."

I was having trouble digesting all this new information. "That explains a lot," I said finally.

"Glen even moved back into that same house when he started working here," Ben said.

"Do you know where that house is?" I said, jumping to my feet.

"Of course I do, sir," Ben said.

My mind was flying again. "Why didn't you tell me you knew?" I said impatiently as Ben scrawled the address on a scrap of paper.

"You never asked me, sir," Ben said as I flew out of the room. "My best to the boy," he called out behind me.

II

The ghetto isn't something you see; it's something you experience. It takes all five senses to draw the place in. I'd driven in and out of the ghetto every day since I'd come to The Bin, but that's all it had been—in and out. I'd always gone on the main roads with the best lighting. So I'd never really been "in" the ghetto. Never driven down the side streets peering for an address. I'd never had business there. Until the night I set out to find Glen Charles. Until I actually drove into the heart of darkness.

There are many things I could say about my feelings and impressions from that evening. I could tell you how appalled I was. How frightened. How angry. But I won't. Instead, I'll tell you a ghetto story.

Not far from Glen Charles's home, I pulled up to a red light. There was a naked man in the intersection, obviously confused and dazed. PCP was my guess. A car pulled alongside me and the driver got out. He walked up to the naked man and punched him in the face, knocking him to the ground. Then he got back in his car. As soon as the fellow in the intersection had struggled to his feet, a second man from a car across the way also punched him to the pavement. Then the light changed and we all drove off. I know this story means something; I just don't know what it is.

After a little difficulty, I located the house number Ben had given me. The small, two-story structure was in the middle of a block of similar homes, all in a final struggle against total delapidation.

For every sidewalk fence that was standing, one was sagging over.

Spray-painted gang slogans were winning the battle to wash them away. Boards were replacing windows. Even the grass was dying.

I quickly pulled to the curb, checked my address again, and got out of the car. On the sidewalk in front of Glen's house, I had another pang of indecision. I felt I was violating his territory. That I was somewhere I shouldn't have been. I think I was just plain scared about where I was and what I might find. But then I remembered what Ben had said. Taking a deep breath, I opened the small chain-link gate and walked up to the door.

The house was completely dark. The only sound was a siren in the distance. I checked Ben's address a third time, then knocked on the door. The sound echoed in my ears like artillery fire. I knocked again. Still nothing. Instinctively, I tried the handle. It wasn't locked.

That's when my last personal crisis came. I stepped back and looked up at the house. I was paralyzed. As I stood breathing that thick night air, I turned and gazed up and down the street. Suddenly, I could see Glen Charles as a boy playing there, hitting baseballs, riding a bike, laughing. Then I looked at the houses nearby and the lights in the distance.

A speeding car jarred me from my reverie. Music blaring, a long red convertible zoomed past the house and screeched around the corner. I turned around again to face the door. Glen had survived all this, I thought; he wasn't going to blow it now. I walked inside.

The house was black as pitch and silent as a tomb. But somehow I knew I wasn't alone. That little voice in my head was screaming too loud.

Nervously edging my way forward, I peered into the darkness. As I gradually became accustomed to the black, I began to make out some dim outlines, a chair here, a table there. I heard a clock ticking. Then I saw the stairs.

I crept over and stared toward the landing on top. I was about to call out when the whole house shook from what I first thought was a clap of thunder. Then I realized it was a shotgun blast.

"Glen!" I screamed and blindly charged upstairs. I stopped in my tracks on the second floor. The sound was muffled at first but it eventually became more distinct. Someone was crying.

I reached out and slowly swung open the door in front of me. Silhouetted in gray window light, Glen Charles was sitting on the edge of his bed, his face in his hands. There was a rifle at his feet. The room smelled of spent gun powder.

I think Glen knew I was there, but neither of us spoke or moved. I couldn't take my eyes off him. I'm haunted to this day by the depth and pain of his sobs. Then that strange calmness came back over me and I walked in.

I picked the gun off the floor and quickly flung it out of reach. The barrel was still warm. Broken glass crunched under my feet from the shattered mirror above Glen's dresser. It had obviously taken the brunt of the blast.

On top of the bureau, amid the shards of smashed glass and splintered wood, I lifted out a torn bit of paper that I held up to the window. It was half of an old photograph. I recognized the face. It was Glen Charles—only older. It was a picture of his father.

Finally Glen took a breath and wiped his face. "I couldn't do it," he moaned. "I can't even shoot myself right. My father had me pegged."

I walked over and put my hand on Glen's shoulder. "Your father's dead," I said slowly. "You don't have to please him any more."

Glen was still breathing hard. "That damned old man . . ." he said, sniffing and shaking his head. His hands were trembling like leaves.

"Ben says he was a real son of a bitch," I said, not knowing what Glen's response would be.

Glen clasped his hands together. A small light outside the window was glistening off his wet, tear-stained face. He stared at me for the longest time. "You know about Ben?" he finally mumbled.

"Yes, I do," I replied. "And I think he's a pretty good judge of character."

Then we were both silent again for what seemed like an hour. My hand never left Glen's shoulder. Gradually, finally, he seemed to calm a little. Then he shuddered and I realized it was a laugh. "I really blew the shit out of him, didn't I?" Glen said, taking the small scrap of picture from my hand.

"Long overdue if you ask me," I said.

Glen looked back at the picture. Then there was another long pause. "I agree," he said evenly.

I gave Glen a chance to get himself together. Then we walked down the stairs. "You'll stay with us tonight," I said.

"I'll be okay now, really," Glen said, begging off.

Along with the picture of his father, that shotgun blast had also at last blown away Glen's burdensome Dr. Charles image. "You're my friend," I said firmly. "You'll stay with us."

Glen thought for a moment, then offered his hand. "Thanks," he said. "I'd like that."

I took Glen's hand in both of mine. "Welcome to the human race," I said quietly.

Glen was quiet during the thirty-minute freeway drive to my house. He rolled down the passenger-side window, closed his eyes, and leaned his head into the breeze.

"We're here," I said, finally pulling up our drive.

Glen sat up slowly and looked around. Then he looked at me and smiled. Side by side we strode up the walk and in through the front door.

It was late. My wife and kids were already in bed and I decided not to disturb them. There would be time for explanations in the morning. I wrapped my bruised hand in ice, then Glen and I ate warmed-up leftovers and talked into the night. Really talked. I convinced him to enter therapy, at least for a while. It was, as they say, the beginning of a beautiful friendship.

Glen was a little quiet for a few days at work. No explanations were asked for and none were given. Things were gradually just allowed to settle back to normal. Thinking back on all that happened, you really had to admire the guy. Which, I believe, is where I started about Glen Charles.

III

I had a varied group of patients that winter. And lots of them. We hadn't had an empty bed for months. When winter sets in back East, the ranks of L.A.'s homeless swell. Sleeping in a Minneapolis park loses some of its luster when it's ten below outside. As February drew to a close and the promise of spring was in the air, I thought back on the past few months.

I'd cared for a continual array of schizophrenics, those poor souls lost in a sea of suspicion, doubt, and despair. There were cocaine addicts who couldn't climb out of their post-drug crash. PCP users who'd plucked out an eye or jumped from a building or severed an appendage. The drinkers' convulsion and trembling through withdrawal. The manics. The depressives. The borderlines. I'd treated, it seemed, an entire legion of wretched and tormented souls. There was one notable bright spot, however.

Just after New Year's, Mr. Aziz, the rug merchant, finally slowed down and we were able to talk. "What do you mean I gave all my money away?" he said after I thought he was strong enough to handle the news.

"You took it from the bank and threw it out the car window," I said. "Down on Crenshaw Boulevard."

Mr. Aziz looked at me in a strange, hopeful way. "This is a joke, right?" he said, forcing a smile. "An American doctor joke?"

When I assured the man I wasn't kidding, Mr. Aziz went into some kind of trance. "Twenty years," he mumbled over and over. After ten minutes of this I became a little worried. Then he seemed to snap back for a while. "Does my wife know?" he asked.

"I'm afraid she does," I replied.

"How'd she take it?" Mr. Aziz asked, looking like he already knew the answer.

I remembered back to that first night when the whole Aziz clan had come to visit. When they only knew that Mr. Aziz was in a mental hospital but didn't know why. I remembered how many of us it took to subdue Mrs. Aziz when she first heard what happened. "I'll kill that lunatic with my bare hands," she shrieked, trying to claw her way toward her husband.

Abdul Aziz was the only patient I saw all year that I could guarantee would take his medication. After I explained to him and his wife that the only way to prevent a recurrence of his symptoms was to stay on the lithium, Mrs. Aziz gave Mr. Aziz a long stare.

"I'll take it," Mr. Aziz said nervously. "I'll eat it. I'll bathe in it. Anything." Then he glanced back at his wife who was still staring at him.

Mae Peterson had been discharged in mid-January. She said she was feeling better. I knew she was eating better and her sleep was undisturbed. She went back out to her board-and-care home.

Before she left I showed her the watch she'd given me. It was under a small glass dome on my desk. She smiled a long, slow smile but didn't say anything. She didn't have to.

I was still uncomfortable with Ricky Myers, but now for different reasons. Things were going too well. The gains he'd made over the holidays were maintained and then some. He began to participate in ward activities, and I found him actually engaging other patients in casual conversation.

He was drawn to Mae Peterson for a while and, oddly, she didn't seem to mind. The two frequently spent evenings chatting in the dayroom while watching TV. Ricky still appeared a little uncomfortable with conversation, but much less so than before. Mae seemed to be good for him, something, I had to admit, I hadn't really been. But watching those two gave me a shiver. Ricky Myers looked so damn normal. At times I even had to remind myself of Minnie Osbourne's words. The man talking so amiably with Mae Peterson was, at the core, a bad happening.

And our sessions together had even become semi-productive, although somewhat repetitive. For his part, Myers seemed to enjoy talking about his childhood—he'd played baseball, something we shared in common—while I spent my time emphasizing over and over the importance of his continuing to take his medication.

Things were going so well, in fact, that Ricky Myers actually began to blend in. People stopped looking over their shoulder whenever he was around. I hadn't pressed administration to hurry his transfer in weeks. His killings were rarely mentioned anymore. We all stopped worrying. And our guard slowly slipped down. One morning I saw Dr. Singh actually touch Myers on the shoulder as they passed in the hallway.

It was weird, I found, how things on the ward tended to run in cycles. One month, it seemed, the majority of our patients would be schizophrenics. Then we would get a bunch of bipolars or a group of depressives. We rarely had a stranger month than March, however, when three of our patients were pregnant and one only thought so.

Kay Lyle, Bertha Beamon, and Sheena Carlysle were all admitted within a week of each other. All were in their last trimester. Bob

Hurley, the man who believed he was pregnant, was definitely full term.

Delusions, as I said, are beliefs impervious to reason. How or why they happen is anyone's guess. But they are very real. People just get an idea in their head and won't let it go. In some, but not all cases, medication will break the logjam.

Delusions are not limited to any specific psychiatric diagnosis. They cut across all borders. They come in different types as well. Bipolars' delusions tend to be grandiose. People like Mr. Aziz believe they are millionaires. The man who thinks he's Napoleon is a classic example.

Schizophrenics' delusions tend to be bizarre or paranoid. They might say the CIA is controlling them with space beams, or a flock of chickens lives in their stomach. The delusions of severe depression run on the more morbid side. "My brain is rotting," one patient told me.

The problem with delusions goes back to their definition. People really believe them and, as such, run their lives accordingly. Napoleon may wander onto an army base and start barking orders. When the beams get too intense, a paranoid might plant a bomb at a government building. Or a depressive could take a gun to his head to let out the rot.

And, strangely, sometimes a person's body actually goes along with the program. Mr. Hurley was admitted through triage after the police were called to a local Lamaze center where he'd repeatedly presented himself for childbirth classes. When I first saw him I was dumbfounded. He actually looked pregnant. His breasts were enlarged. His hips had spread. And he had the waddle down pat. It took him forever to get in and out of a chair.

Medication during pregnancy is always a thorny issue but never more so than with psychiatric drugs. Most of our medicines have known effects on a growing fetus, some of which are potentially disastrous. Antipsychotic drugs, Thorazine and the like, cause muscle-tone problems after birth. The antianxiety group, Valium, etc., may lead to cleft palates. Lithium exposure in utero is linked to heart-valve defects.

So, as the common medical axiom goes, the risks must be weighed against any potential benefits. In other words, is it safer for a child to be exposed to drugs or have a crazy mother? Each case is different. The final decision is never an easy call.

Here's how things were laid out for us and our four pregnancies. Bob Hurley got medication. Kay Lyle, a young woman of twenty in the middle of her second schizophrenic break, did not. Kay's delusions were peculiar but not, we felt, potentially harmful. She had a tiny bird in her head that spoke to her in whistles, which is also how Kay spoke back. We all hoped Kay's baby appreciated what we were doing for it. For a month Ward Three sounded like an aviary.

Bertha Beamon, thirty-four with five children already, didn't get medicine, either. Bertha was a Bin regular. In the past, she'd never responded very well to drug treatment, so we saw no pressing reason to try again. Bertha heard voices telling her to turn on the shower and stove. At home this could be a nightmare. In the hospital it was manageable.

Sheena Carlysle was the problem. Sheena, an attractive black woman of thirty-three, was having a manic break. The trouble was this: Sheena Carlysle desperately wanted that baby, having miscarried twice before. She was in the middle of her eighth month. She'd never carried a child this long. This, she was convinced, was the one.

Mania comes in two kinds, euphoric and crabby. It's important to distinguish between the two because treatments may vary. Sheena had the happy kind. Unfortunately, she also had the busy kind. She was running on fast forward twenty-four hours a day. If she kept up her pace much longer, we knew, she would collapse. And if she didn't die, surely the baby would.

After lots of discussion, I began Sheena on lithium, and Klonopin with Ativan (a short-acting sedative) injections if she really got out of hand.

Then for the next month throughout March, it seemed, all we did was hold our breath. We all liked Sheena Carlysle a lot. We liked her husband. We were really rooting for that baby.

As Sheena's delivery date, March twenty-third, drew near, our spirits soared. Mother was under control and baby seemed to be doing fine. Everyone had their fingers crossed. Things looked good.

Then The Accountant struck. The great leveler. If we were going to receive a precious gift, something equally precious would have to be taken in return.

"I found these pills hidden under Ricky Myers's mattress," Ben Smith said to me the morning Sheena Carlysle had her first labor pain.

EIGHTEEN

AMAZING GRACE

I

SCHIZOPHRENIA IS AN unusually awful disease. One percent of the U.S. population has it. That's about 2,500,000 people or roughly the population of Idaho, Utah, and Nevada combined. This one percent figure remains fairly stable throughout the world, in fact. No ethnicity or geographic location is spared. There are five billion people in the world. You figure it out.

Schizophrenia is an inherited disorder. It runs in families. It's not caused by bad mothering. It doesn't mean split personality. The disease, so holds current theory, is a problem with dopamine transmission in the brain. Dopamine is one of the body's many neurotransmitters. Neurotransmitters are chemicals that brain cells, neurons, use to communicate with one another.

When a person's dopamine network goes haywire, they develop the symptoms of schizophrenia. Their brain is either sending or receiving the wrong message. That's why schizophrenics are so bizarre. Their head wiring's all tangled up. They hear voices when no one is speaking. They believe unusual things. They have trouble forming a coherent sentence. They forget to bathe and shave. Understandably, this makes normal social intercourse a difficult proposition. It's terrifying just to think about.

Schizophrenics fall into five basic categories: catatonic, disorganized, paranoid, residual, and undifferentiated. At the turn of the century when we were a more peaceful, agrarian society, the majority of schizophrenics were catatonic. Catatonia basically means a disorder of movement or posture, either too much or too little. These are people who will strike a pose and hold it for weeks or become so excited they die from exhaustion. You don't see much of this any more.

Carl Williams was a disorganized schizophrenic. These people, as I said, have a silly quality to them. Residual schizophrenics are people who slowly dissolve into total apathy without ever experiencing the usual symptoms of a "nervous breakdown." They don't hear voices. They don't think they're God. Their minds just slowly crumble away. Undifferentiated schizophrenics, the majority, don't fall into any of the other classifications. A good percentage of the homeless population suffer from this form of the disease.

Paranoid schizophrenics, the final category, are a different matter altogether. They may, in fact, have an entirely different disease. Many paranoid schizophrenics work and have families. Some, in fact, get along quite well. They do, unfortunately, suffer from delusions and occasionally hear voices.

Paranoid schizophrenics think people or things are out to get them. The FBI follows them. The CIA has their phone tapped. Aliens talk to them through phone wires. As our society has become increasingly more complex and technologically sophisticated, the number of paranoid schizophrenics has increased proportionally, which, if you think about it, makes sense in a strange sort of way.

The voices these people hear are different, too. The voices tell them who is after them and why. The voices often take the form of God or Satan. The voices tell these people to do things. Like barricade themselves in an office. Or buy automatic firearms. Or kill. And every so often these people obey.

II

Rounds began that late March morning at nine on the dot. Whatever could be said of Dr. Singh, our chief, he was orderly in his thinking and in his life. I admired the man a great deal. He'd taught me so much. He was always in control, always on top of things. There was never a hair out of place in his beard or even the smallest wrinkle in his clothes. "Are there any new patients?" he said that morning as he sat at the head of the assembled staff.

It was all just luck of the draw, really. One of those random events that eats at your yearning for universal certainty. It's like getting struck by lightning, I guess. I mean, why was someone at that spot at exactly that moment? Chance is a difficult thing to deal with, especially when it comes to death. Anyone of us could have been the first one out that door.

Rounds lasted an hour and a half, as always. Two new patients were presented and all the old ones discussed. I was asked to explain the mechanism of action for an anti-depressant medication which, gratefully, I had just read up on. Dr. Ashwin expounded on cocaine addiction in her usual gentle and eloquent manner. Glen Charles detailed a research article he'd recently read in a British scientific journal. And our generally stodgy psychologist, Dr. Lamb, ended by telling a joke. He recited a small verse he'd read in a magazine. "Roses are red, Violets are blue, I'm schizophrenic, And so am I," he said, and we all laughed, especially Miss Givens who, for some reason, found the poem particularly funny.

"I'm late for a staff meeting," Dr. Singh said finally, standing to leave. "If you have any problems, page me." Then he walked out of the room.

"I said we'll talk later, Ricky," we heard him say from the hall. "You'll have to excuse me now. I'm in a hurry." I imagined there was just time for him to turn his back.

You could hear the bones crack. There was no shouting. No sounds of a scuffle. Just the repeated blows of hard metal against Dr. Singh's skull.

By the time we all scrambled outside it was over. Two burly attendants had Ricky Myers pinned to the floor. He wasn't struggling. His mission was accomplished. "Die, Satan! Die, Satan!" he was screaming over and over again. White spittle was frothing at the corners of his mouth.

The staff was absolutely silent. We were all simply overwhelmed. Everyone backed away in an ever-widening circle as if, somehow, distancing yourself from the horror would make it less real.

At the center of this terrified ring of staggering people a folding chair lay flat on the tile. On an outer edge, the part that had sliced through Dr. Singh's head, were two tufts of black hair and a thick red streak of clotting blood.

Dr. Singh lay motionless beside the chair. His arms and legs were splayed apart as if he were swimming. His head was tilted and pushed up against the near wall. His sky-blue turban, now awash with fresh blood, was tipped upside down alongside him like a beggar's cup. "Die, Satan! Die, Satan!" Ricky Myers kept screaming.

Somehow, fortunately, someone had kept their wits and called for help. "Code Red. Ward Three. Psychiatry," came the announcement from the overhead speakers.

The next while was all pretty much of a blur. The initial shock finally wore off and suddenly everyone was shrieking. Two more security guards arrived to manacle Ricky. In a fit of rage one of the nurses began kicking Myers in the back. She had to be pulled away.

I remember the hall was packed with people. I remember IV lines and medicines and screaming and reaching. I remember seeing faces from the outside corridor crowding the small ward door window. I remember Dr. Ashwin backed against a corridor wall standing absolutely motionless. I remember Miss Givens's frantic voice shouting for people to move back. I remember Glen Charles and I alternately pumping on Dr. Singh's chest. I remember hearing a doctor I didn't know say, "Let's stop. He's dead." The last thing I remember is promising to kill Ricky Myers.

III

It was March twenty-seventh and a particularly warm day for being just barely spring. The sky was a soft pastel blue. A single crisp white cloud seemed to bounce off the horizon like a child's ball. Above me two birds were softly twittering. For L.A., the air felt surprisingly clean.

I sat on a small bench beneath the trees, spread my arms across the wooden back, and turned my face into the sun. Dr. Ashwin was with me out behind the old maintenance building but she'd sought her own solitude. I watched intently as a small colored moth fluttered down and lit on the toe of my shoe.

Dr. Singh had been buried that morning and no one felt like working. Miss Givens had simply gone home. Dr. Ashwin and I were drawn to our secret garden. Glen Charles was keeping watch on the ward.

Despite working ER for so long and knowing death on such an intimate basis, nothing I'd previously experienced prepared me for the loss of Dr. Singh. Maybe it was the suddenness or how it happened or who did it. I don't know. I just knew it hurt so bad. Ever since that terrible morning four days before, I'd felt like someone had run a sword through me.

I know the rest of the staff was in just as much pain as I. It was the look in everyone's eyes. That stare. A stare of dumbfounded rage and sorrow. We were all shattered.

I had another emotion to work through as well. I'd never hated anything or anybody as much as I hated Ricky Myers right then. I knew my feelings had to be dealt with before they consumed me. I wanted to kill him. I wanted to torture him. I wanted him to feel pain, real pain. I wanted to tear him apart and stomp on the pieces.

After security hauled him away that morning, I never saw Myers again. I didn't care where they took him. I didn't care what happened to him. I just knew that if our paths happened to cross again I couldn't guarantee my actions.

I sat for most of that afternoon out in our garden. Dr. Ashwin stayed as well. I passed the time thinking over the last nine months, remembering all that had happened and especially the many hours I'd spent with Dr. Singh.

I remembered all I'd learned from him. How he'd always set an example of academic integrity and professional conduct. I truly loved and respected the man. I thought about seeing his wife and children at the gravesite. They looked so shocked and empty. I didn't dwell on this last part, however. I wasn't sure how much was left holding me together.

Finally Dr. Ashwin walked up. "We have to go," she said quietly. "There are two new admissions." I nodded and stood. You could see the top of County General above the trees. We both just stared for a moment, then instinctively took each other's hand and headed back.

And slowly, as if driven by some irresistible, unseen force, life on Ward Three began to start up again. The right papers got filled out. Meals came and went. Beds were made and slept in. Somehow we managed to keep going. But something big was missing from our lives and from the ward. Something that could never be replaced.

For two weeks we all seemed to be just going through the motions. We still met for rounds on Monday, Wednesday, and Friday mornings but, even with Glen Charles in charge, the sessions were listless and perfunctory. The essentials of patient care were discussed and that was it. We were all cowed by the sad sight of that empty chair at the head of the conference room table. We were truly a crew that had lost their captain.

The one image I recall most vividly from that awful time is finding myself standing in the corridor one afternoon casually checking a patient's chart. It was late. The hallway was empty. After a while, I happened to glance at the floor. There on the yellow tile, just beside my right shoe, was a tiny dark speck. I stared until the pain overwhelmed me and I had to walk away. The speck on the floor was a tiny dot of Dr. Singh's blood the cleanup crew had missed.

That was the low point for me. Such a beautiful, articulate man reduced to a speck on the floor. I sat in my office a good long time after that. I didn't cry. Strangely, I recalled, leaning back in my chair, I had seen very few people actually cry over the loss of Dr. Singh. I was simply beyond crying and I think the others were, too. I knew I would have to heal a little first before I was capable of tears.

And, of course, everyone's feelings aside, the patients' lives continued on.

Bob Hurley responded to medication nicely. His pregnancy decelerated until it was gone. Then he went back to his family. I saw him working behind the counter of a sidewalk newsstand two months later. I bought a paper, but he didn't recognize me.

Kay Lyle, whistling all the way, brought her baby to term and had a fine, healthy girl. The child went home with grandmother. Kay came back to the ward. We began her on Haldol and the whistling slowed down a little. A week after Dr. Singh's death, a bed came open on Ward Two and Bertha Beamon was transferred there. Which left Sheena Carlysle.

Sheena's story had a true Ward Three flavor to it. Like I said, she began to have pains on that fateful morning. Then, of course, all hell broke loose. The police came, as did scores of security guards and dozens of frightened onlookers. By the time Dr. Singh's body was finally wheeled away, the place looked like Grand Central Station.

Statements were taken. Pictures snapped. Evidence gathered. Those who'd fainted were given seats in the hall. The weeping were comforted. The angry restrained. And then for the first time in hours, it seemed, there was a moment of quiet.

That's when the baby let out a cry. I looked at Miss Givens. Miss Givens looked at Dr. Ashwin. And Dr. Ashwin looked back at me. Instantly we were all running down the hall.

"It's a boy," Glen Charles said as we skidded to a stop at Sheena Carlysle's door. In his arms he had a small wriggling bundle wrapped with a hospital towel. Sheena had the exhausted, ecstatic look of new motherhood on her face.

It was a real moment. We all stood motionless as Glen Charles gently laid Sheena's baby next to her tear-glistened face where it began to coo contentedly. Behind us police radios were crackling and men with chalk were drawing outlines on the floor.

IV

Two weeks to the day after Dr. Singh's funeral, after a fortnight of rudderless drifting, we got the word: a new attending was coming to Ward Three.

At nine sharp on that morning in early April we were all seated around the conference table as usual. That, however, would prove to be the only usual thing about rounds.

For a few minutes we all fidgeted uncomfortably.

"Weren't we supposed to get a new chief today?" Dr. Ashwin asked, staring toward the empty seat at the head of the table.

"That's what I heard," I said. Resident scuttlebutt had it that someone new from the outside was coming in.

"Anyone know this guy?" Glen Charles said and got blank looks in return.

Miss Givens riffled through a stack of papers in front of her. "Says here his name is Fred Markham," she said, reading from a memo. "Doesn't ring a bell with me."

"Perhaps he can't read a clock," Dr. Lamb said condescendingly, holding his watch to his ear. And he wasn't too far wrong.

"Let's start anyway," Dr. Charles said finally. "If he shows, he shows."

So rounds began. At nine-thirty, midway through discussion of our fourth patient, the door opened. It was Dr. Fred Markham, a thin black man wearing tan corduroy pants, a red polo shirt, and slip-on loafer shoes with no socks.

"Sorry, guys," he said, smiling a broad grin as his marathon-runner lanky frame eased into the room. "I never was much for time."

Slicking back his cornrowed hair that he'd tied in back into a small ponytail, Dr. Markham went around the table and shook everyone's hand, calling us each by our first name.

"Nice to see you, Steve," he said when my turn came. "I'm Fred Markham." Then he looked at my name tag. "Intern, huh?" he added. "Bummer."

For the next hour none of us knew how to act or what to say. It was an extremely disconcerting experience. Each time we addressed our new boss as "Doctor Markham," we were quickly corrected. "Fred, man," he said. "Just Fred." This must have happened fifty times.

And every time a patient was presented, he'd ask the strangest questions. "Tell me something about yourself," he said after Dr. Ashwin had updated us on Kay Lyle.

"I'm sorry?" Anita stammered.

"Tell me something about yourself, about you," Dr. Markham persisted.

Dr. Ashwin shot a quick, pleading glance at me. I just shrugged a little and flicked my eyebrows. I was as confused as she was.

So Dr. Ashwin gave a short, resume-style summation of her life, real vital-statistics stuff.

"No, man," Dr. Markham, Fred, said when she was done. "I want to know about you. What excites you? What do you find exhilarating? What makes you soar?"

Dr. Ashwin looked like she'd just met a man from Mars. I think she wanted to speak but couldn't make her mouth move. "I like to read," she managed to stammer weakly.

"Good, that's a start," Dr. Markham said with a genuine smile. "Next case."

Now Dr. Ashwin was sputtering like an engine. "But . . . but . . . but," she said.

"But what, Anita?" Dr. Markham said sincerely.

"But what about her medications, her lab values?" Dr. Ashwin blurted. This stuff had been our standard grist for the mill all these months.

"Do you want to talk about medicines and lab values?" Dr. Markham asked.

"I think I do," Dr. Ashwin said meekly, and I couldn't help but let out a quiet laugh. Obviously upset, Anita whirled toward me and glared.

"No sweat, Anita," Dr. Markham said calmly. "Laughing is good. It's fun. You can never laugh enough in your life."

Dr. Ashwin didn't know where to look or what to say. She was truly befuddled. "Miss Lyle's labs and medications," Dr. Markham prompted her.

"Prolixin 5 mg BID," Anita said in a dazed, monotone voice. "CBC normal. Repeat thyroid panel normal."

"Are you comfortable with that?" Dr. Markham asked.

"Yes, sir," Dr. Ashwin said finally.

"Fred."

"Yes, Fred."

"Fine."

Incredibly, the whole hour went just like that. Dr. Markham asked Glen Charles if he could sing.

"A little," Glen replied.

"Would you care to sing for us now?" Dr. Markham asked. "I'd like that very much."

I'd never seen Glen Charles embarrassed before. "Maybe next time," he managed to sputter.

"Great!" Dr. Markham said enthusiastically. "We'll look forward to it."

He asked Miss Givens to describe her grandparents. He had me tell him a riddle. He had us all sit quietly and just breathe. Then it was over. "Later, guys," Dr. Markham said after we were done breathing. And he left the room.

No one spoke for a while. Finally Miss Givens broke the spell. "What the hell was that?" she said honestly.

Glen Charles leaned back in his chair. "Ladies and gentlemen," he said, "I believe that was rounds."

After a while we realized Glen was right. Then like survivors of a boat wreck we straggled out of the conference room and into the hall.

Despite the recent loss of Dr. Singh, Dr. Markham quickly became our main topic of conversation. As Dr. Charles, Dr. Ashwin, and I sat down to lunch in the cafeteria that afternoon, he was all we could talk about.

"I don't know if I can handle much more of this," Dr. Ashwin said, ignoring her food and turning toward us. "I've never been so . . . so . . . I don't know what."

She and I were on the same wavelength. "I think he's trying to tell us something," I said. "I just don't know what."

"I think he's trying to tell us he's a Goddamned lunatic," Dr. Ashwin said angrily. I'd never heard her swear before.

"Neither of you have it as bad as I do," Glen Charles added with a smile. "I've got to go home and work up a song for tomorrow."

We were joined by Jeff Farrell, a fourth-year resident like Glen. He looked like the cat that ate the mouse.

"So how's Doctor Markham?" he said mischievously. "I'll bet he's a real trip," he added when none of us could formulate an answer.

"He's no stranger to LSD," I said finally.

Glen Charles eyed Dr. Farrell from a cocked head. "You know this guy?" he asked.

"Sure do," Dr. Farrell said, reaching for the salt. "Has he had anyone sing yet?"

For the next twenty minutes Dr. Farrell had a captive audience. We were like kids around a campfire listening to ghost stories. After the tale was over, however, things made a bit more sense.

Remarkably, Dr. Markham was only five years older than myself. I would have believed ten in either direction. He had a smooth, ethereal quality about him that made age a question you never thought to ask. And his credentials were impeccable. Undergrad, University of Pennsylvania. Medicine, UCSF class of '71. Residency at Stanford. When we added up the dates, however, there was a two year gap. "Nam," Dr. Farrell said glibly. "101st airborne."

There have been in the history of psychiatry various movements, or schools of thought, that have, in their time, held sway. Some stayed. Most went as quickly as they'd come.

The first and most lasting revolution was, of course, psycho-analysis. In the early years of the century, Sigmund Freud's painstaking observations and brilliant, synthetic technique opened up the world of the unconscious mind.

Freud's vehicle into this previously unknown world was free association (say anything and everything that comes to mind) and analysis of transference, those strange, unexplained emotions a patient thrusts upon his therapist. His psychic mechanics and dynamic techniques still form the backbone of therapy today.

To be certain, there are other explanations for human action and motivation than those supplied by Freud. Learning theory states that we just repeat reinforced behaviours through a reward and punishment system. Behaviour theorists claim we act more in response to our environment than any internal drive. Each explanation has its proponents and detractors.

There have been a few odd postulations along the way as well. Wilhelm Reich, one of Freud's earliest cohorts, developed a theory of illness and health that involved "orgone," a mysterious cosmic energy. When he, however, began building "orgone energy accumulators" and using them on patients with diagnoses as divergent as schizophrenia and cancer, the FDA stepped in. The theory of "orgone" died when Reich passed away in prison.

In more recent times, the push has been for advances in group therapy as a means for self-exploration. There are three basic types of group treatment.

First are support groups, usually people with the same type of problem who meet to share ideas, let off steam, and prop each other up. The twelve-step programs of AA and Narcotics Anonymous fall in here. Second are true psychotherapy groups where the goal is not support but insight and change. And finally, in the sixties and seventies, there was one other type of group—the encounter group. That's where Dr. Markham fits in.

The stated goal of encounter groups was increased personal knowledge and awareness, to push, as it were, the edges of one's psychological envelope. Numerous centers sprung up that employed encounter-group principles—Esalen, EST, etc. Some places tolerated psychedelic drug use. Others advocated nudity, ultralong sessions, fasting, etc. It was the golden age of hot tub psychiatry.

Over the years, however, the encounter-group movement slowly fizzled out. Whatever gains people made tended to be short-lived and some persons were actually scarred. To its credit, encounter-group leaders did break some new therapeutic ground and introduced a fresh, freer perspective toward therapy.

"Markham was big in the encounter-group movement," Dr. Farrell said. "I went to a few of his sessions during college. It was pretty wild stuff."

"We know," Dr. Ashwin sighed.

"Stick with him for a while," Dr. Farrell hastened to add. "The man's no fool. You'll eventually see where he's headed." From what I could tell, Dr. Farrell seemed serious.

V

The next morning we were all assembled in the conference room at nine sharp, old habits being hard to break. This time, however, there was no push to begin. We all just sat nervously waiting. Glen Charles was drumming his fingers on the table. I felt like we were about to take a big exam.

"Wonderful morning, isn't it?" Dr. Markham said as he blew into the room at nine-twenty. "Morning's my favorite time of day." We all smiled and nodded. Dr. Charles's drumming grew louder.

"We have a new patient," Dr. Ashwin volunteered after Dr. Markham sat silently at the head of the table for two minutes solid. I was grateful that Anita had chosen to speak. The room was so tense we were all about to burst.

"A new patient. That's tragic," Dr. Markham said sadly. Then he fell silent again.

"Pardon me?" Dr. Ashwin said at last.

"Mental illness is always tragic," Dr. Markham stated. "And especially so when a person has to be hospitalized. We all got to enjoy this fine morning and he didn't. I'm honestly sorry."

I had to admit, I'd never really looked at things in quite that way before. I caught Dr. Charles kind of staring and thinking, too.

"Since we've all started the day with some bad news," Dr. Markham said, "let's balance it with something good." He offered his hand to me across the table. "Take the hand of the person next to you," he said, "and tell them you like them."

Dr. Markham took my hand. "Good morning, Steve," he said. "I like you."

"Good morning, Fred," I stuttered after a moment's hesitation. "I like you, too." And the strange thing is I think I meant it.

Surprisingly, after we'd all shaken hands, rounds almost resembled rounds. We actually discussed a few patients, debated a diagnosis or two, and mentioned some medications. Things were comfortable again. I knew it couldn't last.

We'd waded through half the charts when Dr. Markham turned to Glen Charles. "How do you feel about that song you promised us?" he said. I had to close my eyes. This stuff was killing me.

When I opened my eyes again, Glen Charles was still contemplating. Then he smiled. "Sure, why not," he said. I was convinced that Dr. Markham had long since gone off the deep end and now, it seemed, Glen Charles was about to jump in right behind him.

Then the strangest thing happened. Glen actually began to sing. In a slow, low voice he sang the opening verse of "Amazing Grace."

The fact that Glen sang wasn't the strange part. My reaction to it was. I was suddenly overcome with a rush of unexplained sensation. It was like the feeling you got as a kid when they played the Star-Spangled Banner. Or when you first fell in love. I couldn't describe it, but it crashed over me like a big, curling wave. I had to blink to keep from crying.

I know everyone else was just as touched as I was. Miss Givens had to turn her head and dab her eyes. Even Dr. Lamb obviously had a lump in his throat. A single tear rolled down Dr. Ashwin's cheek.

Dr. Markham let us savor the moment before speaking. "That, folks, is what's known as emotion," he said quietly. "That's what we deal with as psychiatrists. How can we ever understand what our patients are experiencing if we don't understand what we're feeling ourselves?"

"This is where our patients live," Dr. Markham continued. "In this crazy, scrambled world of emotion. Every single person out there," he said, pointing to the door, "is feeling pain or despair or hopelessness. Ask yourself: How can you as their doctors get in touch with those feelings? How can you connect? How can you help relieve that suffering? Because if you can't," Dr. Markham concluded in almost a whisper, "all the medicine in the world will never make them well."

It was one of those turning-point mornings.

NINETEEN

THE BABY MAN

I

WE GOT TO SEE Dr. Markham in action that same afternoon. At the request of all of us, he interviewed Dr. Ashwin's new patient. My opinion of our new attending had gone from open scorn to wild curiosity. I can't remember when I'd looked forward to something more.

Harrison Roosevelt was, by my previous standards, your basic schizophrenic, the kind of patient who generated interesting discussions about dopamine receptors, but not much else. I'd had dozens just like him. Some had gotten better, some hadn't. They were all just a blur of similar stories: hearing voices, Haldol, and board-and-care homes. I'd treated all these people but I hadn't really known them. I didn't think it was possible to know them. I found out different.

Dr. Markham, it seemed, broke all the rules I'd learned about classic interview technique. He left his chair to pace the floor. He gazed out the window. He laughed. He touched the patient. He glossed over most of the symptoms I'd really grilled these people on—voices, delusions, etc. Instead of formally testing Mr. Roosevelt's memory, he asked if he was a baseball fan. "I forget," Dr. Markham asked. "Who won the series in 'sixty-nine?"

Say what you will about Dr. Markham's style, it worked. Mr. Roosevelt, that withdrawn, frightened man, blossomed right in front of us. Somehow, Dr. Markham had mined a hidden vestige of personality and teased it out. He'd connected. By the end of the interview the two were talking like old friends. I was astounded.

And so were Drs. Charles and Ashwin. As Mr. Roosevelt stood to leave the small conference room, he shook each of our hands and thanked us. "You're welcome," we all said, but our minds were elsewhere. None of us could take our eyes off Dr. Markham who was sitting quietly in his chair.

"Well?" he said after Mr. Roosevelt was gone.

"I'll sing anytime you want," Dr. Charles said.

"Beethoven makes me soar," Dr. Ashwin added with a smile. I didn't know what to say.

"Every mentally ill person," Dr. Markham said softly, "has a core of sanity no matter how small or how deeply buried. Some may not even realize it's there. It's our job as psychiatrists," he went on, "to find that core and nurture it, to help it grow. Water it like you would a budding flower. That's something of real value you can give your patients."

Dr. Ashwin looked suddenly uncomfortable. Her question was the one I wanted to ask. "Where do medications fit in then?" she said. "What about everything we've learned so far?"

I was feeling her same angst. I'd spent nine months studying brain chemicals, receptors, and metabolic pathways. It was presented as gospel. Now, it seemed, everything had been toppled by a thin black man with a ponytail.

Dr. Markham smiled. "Of course medications are important," he said to our relief. "In fact they're vital and you should know as much about them as possible. Equally important for you to understand, however," he went on, "is that they're not the end-all and be-all for mental illness. Just as insulin is not the end-all and be-all for diabetes."

Then Dr. Markham paused for a response. I knew the man was a top-notch psychiatrist but perhaps, I thought, he was a little hazy on the treatment of diabetes. "I'm not sure I follow," I said hesitantly.

"If a doctor just gives a teenager insulin and sends her home," Dr. Markham continued, "I'll guarantee they're in for a very rocky time of it. Just like the psychiatrist who only gives Thorazine. You may get someone's voices to stop, just like you get a normal blood sugar with insulin, but there are so many other issues involved. How does a patient feel about his medication? Does he see it as a sign of personal weakness or moral failure?" Dr. Markham ran a hand back over his hair and went on. "What does the patient think about you?" he said. "Does he think you're punishing him? Will he get even by noncompliance? How does a sick person fit into the family constellation? Will others sabotage your plan? Do you see where I'm headed?" he asked, and for the first time our answer to any of Dr. Markham's questions was, "Yes."

"Medications remove the roadblocks to therapy," Dr. Markham continued, "just as therapy removes the obstacles to successful medication treatment. The two go hand in hand. They're inseparable." Then he laughed. "And I can tell you from experience," he said. "Learning about medicines is a lot easier than learning to do therapy."

There is a phrase in psychiatry called the "Aha moment." It happens the instant that little light goes on and you get your first glimpse into what's really happening. When Dr. Markham was done speaking, I had one of those moments. I suddenly saw things very clearly. My aha moment was this: *I'd been learning psychiatry for nearly a year and I knew absolutely nothing about it.*

II

As I mentioned, things at The Bin tended to run in cycles. Unfortunately, a few weeks after Dr. Markham's enlightening presentation, the cycle took a definite downturn and, for me, hit rock bottom.

It was late April. The night air was warm and heavy with the feel of the ghetto. It smelled of old men lazing on stoops, cocaine pipes, and crisp dollar bills. It smelled of exhaust from racing and roaring cars. It smelled of broken wine bottles and fluttering napkins stained with fast food. It smelled of life contained, of life stunted, of life struggling and failing to break free.

No air was moving. It was dead calm. There was no moon. I'd just returned from dinner in the main hospital cafeteria and was facing another long night on call when the police car pulled up. Two cops got out and dragged Aaron Johnston from the backseat.

"Get them off me! Get them off me!" Aaron screamed, as the policemen struggled to get him up the ramp and in through our triage area doors.

At first I thought Aaron was talking about the cops but once inside he shouted, "They're crawling up my nose! Please stop them!" He was spinning his head wildly from side to side. His wrists were cuffed behind him.

Finally, as the police began to fill out the necessary hold forms, Aaron Johnston curled up on the tile floor. "Please get them away," he sobbed, drooling and drenched with sweat. Aaron Johnston was seven years old.

III

Aaron Johnston discovered his parents' stash of cocaine and kids, being the great imitators, had decided to try a few lines. Tactile hallucinations, thinking bugs are crawling on you, etc., are common in cocaine ODs. Aaron Johnston screamed for twenty-four hours solid. And I wish I could say that during the year he was the only child I saw like that or that his case was the worst. But neither would be true.

At least Aaron's experience with cocaine had been an accident. Alisha Carmen and Keena Washington weren't so lucky. They were given their drugs on purpose. And they weren't the only ones. Usually the drugs were part of some sexual abuse or cult scenario.

I mentioned the two girls, Alisha and Keena, because they were damaged so badly that gynecological surgery was required. It's very difficult to describe your feelings when you face a ten-year-old girl who's actively hallucinating and bleeding from the vagina. It gives new meaning to the word rage.

I'd planned a detailed account of a case or two of such abuse but, frankly, I found I couldn't do it. The emotions are still too hot, my anger too near the surface. Once begun, I'm afraid I might not stop. I'll have to save it for later. Maybe next time.

Suffice it to say that adults having sex with children is out there— fathers and daughters, fathers and sons, mothers and daughters, mothers and sons, aunts and uncles with nephews and nieces, brothers with sisters, neighbor with neighbor. I thought only animals cannibalized their young.

And, as I found out, we not only have intercourse with our children, sometimes we sell them as well.

I'd just finished placing Aaron Johnston in our padded PES seclusion room when the call came from triage about another patient. "I'll take it," Dr. Lopez, who was working with me, said.

"No way," I replied, standing and heading for the elevator. I needed something to get my mind off Aaron. His screams were still echoing in my head.

As it turned out, I should have listened to Dr. Lopez. The person I went to see was Alice Meacham. Alice was a "strawberry," a woman who trades sex for drugs. When men do it they're called "raspberries."

Alice was a pretty young black woman, thin as a rail and trembling like a leaf.

"I gotta get off this coke, man," she said, sitting in our triage interview room. "It's gonna kill me." Then she shifted slightly. "And I need to get my kids back," she added.

By now, dealing with drug people had become old hat. I'd heard the story over and over: arrest, court, children placed in foster homes. "So what else is new?" I thought to myself. Unfortunately, I found out.

"Where are your kids now?" I asked blandly.

"I sold them," Alice said.

I wasn't certain I'd heard correctly. "You what?" I said, suddenly snapping to and facing forward.

"I sold them. But now I want them back," Alice persisted.

"Who'd you sell them to?" I asked incredulously.

"To the baby man, of course," Alice said.

I was sure I was missing something. I hadn't yet become totally jaded. I was still willing to give people the benefit of the doubt. "I don't understand," I said. "What's a baby man?"

Alice looked a bit irritated. "The baby man is the man who buys babies, children," she said flatly.

I could feel something deep inside me begin to simmer. My gut was getting hotter by the second. Still in a state of total disbelief, I put things to Alice Meacham one more time. "Let's be sure I'm clear," I said carefully. "You gave your children to a man and took money for them?"

"No," Alice said to my momentary relief. "I traded them for cocaine," she continued, and the volcano began to boil.

"You sold your children for crack?" I said in a steely, measured tone.

"Yes," Alice Meacham replied. "I already told you that. Now I need your help to get them back."

"What does this 'baby man' do with the children he buys?" I asked, not daring even to think of the answer.

"I don't know," Alice said, leaning back a little more comfortably. "But it's probably nothing good."

" 'Probably nothing good,' " I repeated slowly. I was on automatic pilot now.

"Well," Miss Meacham said impatiently. "Can you help me?"

Then everything fell into place. I stood up slowly. "We do not do drug detox here," I said, mechanically repeating my standard explanation. "The county won't pay for it. They prefer to spend money on more police and larger jails." I knew the words were coming out correctly but I wasn't sure why. My mind was a million miles from that interview room. I'd gone into total shutdown.

"As far as getting your children back," I said, walking to the door, "no, I won't help you because, frankly, I think you'd just sell them again. But there are lots of people here. Talk with some of them. Who knows." I turned one last time. "Now if you'll excuse me," I said, "I have to go."

I left Alice Meacham sitting on our couch and walked out of the triage area, unlocked the door to Ward Three, and headed for my office. I needed a break. I needed a vacation. I needed something.

As I unlocked the door, a piece of note paper flipped up from the floor. On it was a phone number, beneath which was written "urgent." I recognized Miss Givens's handwriting.

I called the number. It was Martin Braga's mother. She was crying. She said Martin had enrolled in school in Colorado. She said he'd stopped taking his medicine. That morning he'd hung himself in a dormitory stairwell. She said she thought I should know. "Martin liked you," she added, then hung up.

I set the phone down and left my office. "Doctor Seager?" the receptionist called as I passed back through triage and out the door. But I didn't answer. I walked to my car and drove home.

"Don't ask," I said quietly to my startled wife who was just preparing to go to bed. I made straight for the back patio where I slid the glass door closed behind me, pulled up a deck chair, propped my feet on a nearby picnic bench, and stared out into the dark, starry night.

I was half frozen when I woke at dawn, having long since thrown off the blanket my wife had carefully covered me with the night before. I stiffly struggled into the kitchen and made myself a cup of coffee, took one sip, and pitched it into the sink. I've always hated coffee. I made the cup, honestly, because I didn't know what to do with myself.

I didn't know what I was going to do with the remainder of the morning, the afternoon, or the rest of my life for that matter.

At that moment I was only certain of one thing. I was never going back to County General, never going to set foot inside The Bin again. Even if I'd wanted to.

My personal feelings aside, I had broken the cardinal rule of medical training. I'd left a call shift. I'd abandoned my post, slunk away under fire. It's the kind of thing the military shoots people for. The thinking is this: If you desert your patients now, when you have backup, what can we expect when you're on your own?

I checked the clock. It was nearly seven. In two hours everyone at work would know my story. I reached for a magazine and began flipping pages. "Better get used to this," I said to myself.

As I sat with that magazine in my hand, listening to the first stirrings of life in the house around me, I was flooded with images and they were all bad. Martin Braga was dead. Minnie Osbourne was dead. Dr. Singh had been murdered. Ricky Myers was alive. I saw the face of Glen Charles as he wept with a gun at his feet. I saw Big Daddy Benson's face as he smugly tried to slash our meager budget. I heard Aaron Johnston's pathetic wails. And, above it all, two words came over and over again to my mind. They were relentless. They were torturing me. The two words were "baby man."

On his golden wedding anniversary a man was asked about the secret of getting along with a woman for fifty years. "First you have to pick the right woman," was his answer, and I couldn't agree more. I know that's what I did.

"How do you feel?" Linda said, cinching her bathrobe as she padded barefoot into the kitchen.

"Great," I mumbled. "Considering I'm unemployed."

"Rough night?" she said, calmly pouring herself a glass of orange juice.

"You might say that," I replied, setting down my magazine.

"What are you going to do?" she asked.

"Suicide's always an option," I said, then smiled. Suddenly the whole episode seemed too strange to be real.

"You didn't answer my question," Linda persisted.

I was angry and upset. "I don't know what I'm going to do," I snapped. "I left a call shift. I fucked up. They'll fire me for sure."

"Is it something you can talk about?" Linda said, walking over to sit beside me.

"Someday maybe," I said more calmly. "Right now I can't find the words. I don't want to think it's really possible there are such words."

"Do you want to go back?" Linda asked, compassionately changing the subject.

"Yes and no," I said honestly. "Yes, I want to be a psychiatrist. It's the most interesting and worthwhile thing I've ever done." Linda put her hand gently on top of mine. "But I can't handle County General any more. The place is just too much. The issues are too big. Nothing will ever solve them. I need to go someplace where the odds are fair. Where people have a chance in life. Where they're not dead before they're born."

My youngest son walked in the room. In a definite transition phase, he was wearing a Hulk Hogan T-shirt and pajama bottoms printed with ducks. "Morning, Dad," he said, crossing to the refrigerator with a wave.

"Morning," I replied. "Did you sleep well?"

"Right on, dude," he said, disappearing with a cup of milk back into his room.

My wife was silent for a while, but I knew what she was thinking. "I'll go back, at least to apologize," I said finally. "I owe them that."

"I think that's best," Linda said quietly.

It was an agonizing drive back to The Bin. I tried to imagine talking to Dr. Markham and Dr. Jefferson, my supervisor. I tried to visualize the other residents as they heard the news. I tried to imagine how I was going to pay the bills.

Certain of the worst, I headed straight for the PES. I kept some books down there and this was as good a time as any to collect them.

My heart was pounding as I walked through those big sliding doors and into the triage area. I glanced quickly into the small interview room, half expecting to see Alice Meacham still sitting on the couch waiting for me. The room was empty, so I made for the elevator. Taking a breath, I keyed it open and rode downstairs.

I could barely make my feet move; I was seeing all those faces again. That walk around the corner to the nursing station was the longest of my life. At that moment I hated Alice Meacham, I hated County General, and I hated myself. But, thankfully, I thought as I stepped inside to face the music, it would all soon be over.

As I stood among the seated nurses just finishing their shift report,

I was honestly surprised. They just went right on with what they were doing. There were no suspicious stares. No whispered words. Nothing. They didn't, in fact, even seem to notice I was there.

"Oh, Doctor Seager," Gloria Phipps, the night nurse, finally said. "Is everything okay at home?" She seemed more concerned than angry.

"I'm sorry," I said. I was very confused.

"Your wife called last night," Miss Phipps continued. "I hope it was nothing serious."

"No, everything's fine," I said, thinking how much I loved Linda.

"I'm glad," Miss Phipps concluded. "You look like you've had a hard time. Promise me you'll get some sleep tonight."

"I promise," I said.

Miss Phipps turned and walked toward the door. I caught her just going into the hallway. "What happened to Alice Meacham?" I asked. "The lady I saw upstairs."

Miss Phipps's face turned to iron. "Doctor Charles came in and booted her ass out," she said angrily. "You wouldn't believe the story he told us."

"Doctor Charles?" I asked.

"You do need some sleep," Miss Phipps said, smiling again. "He said you called him in."

"Of course," I mumbled, smiling back. I made a mental note to have a dozen roses delivered to my home.

Uncertain what to do, I walked back to our small call room. I needed time to think. When I opened the door Glen Charles was reading at the desk sandwiched between the two twin beds.

"Don't be late for rounds," he said, glancing up.

"Glen . . . I . . . I . . ." I sputtered. How do you thank a guy for saving your life?

Glen turned back to his book. "Welcome to the human race," he said. "We'll talk later."

TWENTY

A SEAT IN THE LIFEBOAT

I

THANKS TO MY WIFE and Glen Charles, the whole terrible episode with Alice Meacham and my leaving call just blew over. I had a chance to come to my senses. Or, more correctly, with a little help I came to my senses.

"The ghetto is a terrible place," Glen said as we sat in his office that morning after rounds. "Everyone who experiences it," he continued, leaning back in the chair behind his desk, "on a real, gut level has exactly the same reaction you did. I had it. We all had it.

"I know the rage, the terror, the sense of criminal injustice," Glen continued. "The place strikes at deep emotions. We deal with the bedrock here on a daily basis. And," he added with a knowing smile, "if you're lucky enough to come from a place where these issues rarely come up, eventually you explode."

I could only smile back. Glen had it right on the button. The main issue in our neighborhood when I was a child had been with whom to trade baseball cards.

"Growing up here," Glen said, "you adapt early or, literally, you die." His eyes grew a bit distant. "You learn to swallow the hate and pain," he said. "And you just keep on swallowing it until you leave or it consumes you.

"You can, as they say," Glen continued, "take the boy out of the ghetto but you can't take the ghetto out of the boy. As you'll discover, now that you've been here, you can never completely shake loose of the place. You never get rid of the guilt."

"Guilt?" I said as Glen paused for a moment.

"That's the part that eats at you," Glen said with a sigh. "It had a lot to do with your reaction last night. I know it had everything to do with mine. You feel guilty for getting away while so many others are left behind. You feel bad because you got a seat in the lifeboat."

I was suddenly getting very uncomfortable. I knew Glen was onto something. "Everything comes to a head," he continued, "when we realize the ghetto exists not because 'they' tolerate it but because we ourselves tolerate it, you and I. This place is like it is because we allow it to be so. That's the conflict," Glen said. "The kernel for the explosion. How can this place be, and why did I permit it? That's a heavy cross to bear."

I felt like running from the room or punching Glen. He'd found a sore spot and was leaning down hard. I think I actually pulled at my shirt collar.

"There is a way out, however," Glen said with a reassuring look. "Since you were part of the problem, you have to become part of the solution. Not the entire solution, just your part."

"What's my part, Glen?" I said, thinking back to the overwhelming rush of emotion I'd felt while driving through the ghetto streets.

"Your part," Glen continued, "is to take it one person at a time. To realize that all these people are human beings. That they weren't always drug addicts, child abusers, or schizophrenics. That they didn't ask for this, just as you didn't ask for the troubles in your life. Do the best you can for each patient that crosses your path and you've done your job. The larger issues here are too much to comprehend.

But the little ones we can handle. And if enough little ones go away, one day so will the big ones."

I sat across from Glen for a long time. I was running a finger aimlessly around my chin and thinking. Everything Glen said was correct. I did feel guilty and angry. I was ashamed that places like our ghetto existed in my lifetime, and that I tolerated others slipping to the depths of degradation. I was angry that people slept outside and ate garbage and stood in traffic babbling. I hated PCP. I hated cocaine. I hated gangs. I hated hookers and drunks and children in rags. Right then I hated the world and everyone in it. This time, however, I decided to do something about it.

"You were planning to quit and never come back, right?" Glen asked finally.

"I was," I replied.

"Was?" Glen said hopefully.

"Was," I stated firmly.

Right then I became part of the solution. I left Glen's office and went to see my new patient.

II

Benny Darling was already up in his room when I met him. Well, at least he was almost there.

I was seated in the nursing station looking at his chart when I first saw Mr. Darling. He was young, mid-twenties, and, for our population, looked surprisingly good. His hair was combed and he was clean shaven. He'd obviously been eating regular meals. I knew immediately what his problem was.

"How long's he been doing that?" I asked Miss Givens who was sitting beside me.

She looked at her watch, then down the hall. "A good half hour," she said, returning to the paperwork in front of her. "I tried everything I could think of. The damn fool just won't go through the door."

I really felt for Benny Darling. He was obviously suffering. He really wanted to get inside that room. But things had to be just right first.

Benny kept repeating the same sequence of events over and over. First he tapped each side of the door frame twelve times, then closed his eyes and mouthed something as if praying. Then he tapped the door frame again in exactly the same spots with exactly the same fingers. Or almost the same spots and very nearly with the same fingers, because each time this elaborate ritual was complete, Benny began to hyperventilate and stare around frantically. Then he'd begin the whole thing again.

Benny Darling suffered from obsessive-compulsive disorder, OCD for short, a disease much more prevalent than previously thought. It works like this. Intrusive thoughts come to a person's mind, generally concerning impending harm to a family member, global disaster, or some such thing. The person doesn't want the thoughts, recognizes them as foreign, yet is powerless to control them. That's where the compulsions come in. The person discovers that by performing a specific ritual in a specific way he can reduce some of the tension. Soon the connection is made that performing the ritual will prevent Grandma from dying and the cycle begins.

OCD can be an extremely disabling disease. It's difficult to hold a job and shower twenty times a day.

There are three basic OCD types: cleaners, checkers, and worriers. Mr. Darling was a checker. Checkers spend all day lining things up, arranging coins, tapping, counting, looking at the stove. Then they spend all night checking to be certain they've done everything right.

OCD generally strikes a younger, better educated group than most mental disorders. Mr. Darling had a Ph.D. in engineering from

224

Berkeley. He'd worked at a major aerospace firm for five years. Then one day the paper clips on his desk didn't look right.

OCD is called "insanity with insight." These people know their behaviour is ridiculous. They understand there's no correlation between their grandmother's health and how many times they shower. But they just can't help it. You have a sense for OCD if you've ever changed your path to keep from walking under a ladder.

When I reached Mr. Darling he was nearly in a frenzy, praying and tapping so hard I thought he might collapse. One method of treatment I'd read about was to physically prevent people from completing their rituals. I decided to give it a test run. I grabbed Mr. Darling in a bear hug and shuffled him into his room. Still, before he finally quieted down, I had to have Miss Givens administer a strong sedative.

While Freud had his explanations for OCD, current thought holds that it's a structural problem, probably relating to pathology in the frontal lobes and basal ganglia, small structures deep in the brain. Fortunately, there is a medication to which it seems to respond. I began Mr. Darling on clomipramine, an antidepressant, that next morning.

It took a week or so, but Benny Darling gradually came around. The praying stopped first. He quit continually arranging his clothes and then going back to rearrange them. He was left with some residual tapping but nothing, he said, he couldn't handle. Two or three drums of the finger would suffice when entering or leaving a room.

Benny Darling came along at just the right time for me. He responded so well to treatment and he was so grateful, I truly had a sense of accomplishment. I felt good again. I got a letter from Mr. Darling six months later. He'd moved to Seattle and gone back to work.

I hadn't changed the world but, as Glen Charles said, I'd made it a better place for one person. For the first time in a while, I knew the feeling of true satisfaction.

In a way we kind of hated to see Benny Darling leave the ward. There hadn't been a magazine or ashtray out of place in the dayroom for days. And it was the only time I could recall that a patient's room was cleaner when he departed than when he arrived.

III

When Benny Darling left Ward Three it was hard for me to comprehend all that had happened over the past weeks and what a tumultuous, difficult time it had been for everyone. It was less than six weeks ago, I mused, when the biggest concern on the ward was the coming of Sheena Carlysle's baby, who, by the way, was doing fine. Miss Givens kept in regular contact with Sheena and her husband since Sheena's discharge two weeks after her delivery. Mother and baby were both well and happy.

The Carlysles had named their son Singer in honor of Dr. Singh, which I found particularly touching. There was a picture of young Singer Carlysle prominently displayed on the nursing station bulletin board.

Those few short weeks in late March, April, and early May had exposed a raw nerve in all of us. It spoke to the fluidity and uncertainty of life. It spoke of one never really being allowed to be comfortable. That nothing could ever truly be counted upon. That there were no guarantees.

These have always been unsettling issues for me anyway, so despite my recent success with Mr. Darling, I was still feeling uneasy that second week in May. I felt detached and disconnected. I knew I needed to get grounded again, to feel my feet once more firmly on the floor.

And for that I knew exactly where to turn. I paid a call on an old friend. It had taken me awhile after Minnie Osbourne's death before I'd felt I was ready to visit her gravesite. But since mid-January I'd gone there on occasion when I was confused or down and needed a little picking up.

I always brought flowers to set beside the small flat marker that read simply "Minnie Osbourne." I generally had to tidy up the site as, apparently in death as in life, there wasn't much of anyone to care for the poor. Satisfied that Minnie's plot was in order, I unfolded a lawn chair on that mild, sunny May afternoon and sat down for a chat.

I had so much to tell Minnie this time that I stayed longer than usual. I told her about Dr. Singh's tragic death and how she'd been right about Ricky Myers, and about the baby man and my leaving call, and about Glen Charles, and what a good wife I had, and finally I told her about Benny Darling and how good I felt about that.

And, of course, Minnie said all the right things. I could hear her voice in my mind as clearly as if she were sitting there beside me. "Did you follow your heart?" she asked.

"Yes, I did," I replied. "Just like you taught me."

"Then," she said quietly, "you've done all you can do. Let the good Lord take care of the rest."

After an hour or so I felt much better. "Thanks for the time, Minnie," I said, refolding my chair and, one last time, sprucing up the flowers near Minnie's headstone. Then I walked back to my car, put the chair in the trunk, and drove away.

I guess things happen for a reason. Fortunately, I'd had my talk with Glen Charles and Minnie Osbourne so my feelings were once again reasonably straight, and I'd been exposed to Dr. Markham so my therapy options had been widened because I had to be fully armed to handle Delia Davis. I needed all my ducks in a row. Every piston had to be firing.

I admitted Delia one night in mid-May. I was on call with Glen

Charles. It was the night I learned Glen had a slightly perverse side to him.

The night began quietly, which occasionally happened at The Bin. Still it was worthy of comment.

"It's nice when things aren't busy," I said to Glen. We were sitting downstairs in the PES dayroom watching TV. I hadn't seen a patient in over an hour. No sooner were my words out, however, than Glen was called to the phone.

I couldn't hear what was being said, but I did watch him through the window as he spoke. His shoulders slumped and his face dropped. He seemed to mouth the word "shit." Then he turned to look at me and visibly brightened. His smile could only be described as sinister.

"There's a patient upstairs I'd like you to see," Glen said casually, walking back into the dayroom.

"I thought you were up," I said, a bit confused.

"I'm pulling rank," Glen replied with that malevolent grin.

My heart sank. "A real teaching case, huh," I said dejectedly.

Glen's smile widened. "You'll learn something alright," he said. "I can guarantee that."

I found out later that Delia Davis was an intern test case. She was in and out of the hospital so much eventually everyone got to care for her. Treating Delia Davis was your rite of passage. Like the American Indians and their gauntlet. Running the gauntlet meant charging between a double row of men while they beat you with clubs. If you were still standing at the end, you were in, a full-fledged member of the tribe. Delia Davis was my psychiatric gauntlet.

IV

The DSM-III-R manual of psychiatric diagnosis has four different areas in which patients are assessed. They are called axes. Each axis describes a separate section of a patient's life that might have some bearing on his functional level. The idea is to give the doctor a more global picture of his patients, taking everything into account.

Axis I is reserved for the major mental disorders—schizophrenia, bipolar disorder, alcohol addiction, etc. Axis II deals with character pathology, those deviations in personality types that are so disturbing. Axis III codes for physical ailments. Axis IV scores from 1 to 6, the level of any immediate stressor in a person's life, 1 being minor and 6 being something like the death of a spouse. There is one final numbered assessment each psychiatric patient receives. This is called Axis V or Global Assessment Score, GAS. It's the doctor's view of how far from normal function a patient is at any given point in time. The scale runs from 1 to 100, with 100 being perfect and 1 near death. Most people on the street run a GAS of 75–80.

I mention this now because Delia Davis was an axis bonanza. She had stuff everywhere. She suffered from bipolar disorder, had a borderline personality structure, was epileptic, and had just lost her husband. Other than that, Mrs. Lincoln, how was the play?

When I walked into triage I was really struck by Delia Davis. First, she must have gone 300–350 pounds easy. And then, of course, she was naked. A policeman had tried to cover her with his jacket. It looked like she was wearing a lobster bib.

I glanced at the two cops who'd somehow managed to handcuff Delia and herd her inside. Rumpled and sweating with hats askew, they looked as if they'd been dragged behind a car.

If they hadn't been so winded, they probably could have given me some history. But I don't think I would have heard it anyway. "GOD

BE PRAISED!!" Delia was shouting at the top of her lungs. "DAM-NATION TO ALL SINNERS! DAMNATION TO ALL SINNERS!" she screamed. Delia was pacing from one end of the triage area to the other, her feet slapping the floor like someone beating a bass drum.

Needless to say, Delia attracted everyone's attention in the waiting room; a dozen wide-eyed souls stood in a single row at the window. "Call security," I said to our startled receptionist. "Call lots of security."

The two cops and I stood back and watched Delia Davis pace and shout until help arrived. "DAMNATION TO ALL SINNERS!" she yelled, as a string of guards finally marched in through the main door.

After an epic struggle, the eight hospital men at last subdued Delia on the floor and got her covered with a sheet.

"Let's get her down and in restraints," I said, and all the guards looked up at me. I think it was just a reflex.

The security people were spared that arduous task, however, be-cause Delia chose that exact moment to have a grand mal seizure. First she stiffened straight as a board and then went into total body spasms. When she finally quit shaking, she'd urinated on the tile.

I must admit to mixed feelings about Delia's seizure. I knew she was very ill so naturally I felt compassion for her plight. On the other hand, however, a convulsion meant she'd have to get checked over in the medical ER. Somehow, I hoped, they'd find a reason to keep her over there.

Of course, I had no such luck. In a few hours, after tests were done and anti-seizure medication given, a heavily sedated Delia Davis returned on a gurney. She was wheeled to the elevator and taken downstairs.

While Delia was gone, I'd had a chance to talk with the cops and read their hold forms. It seems that Delia had begun to heat up about three days ago. She hadn't eaten or slept during that entire span.

Finally, she'd charged out the door of her home, arriving in an agitated state at a local church, managing, somehow, to lose all her clothes in transit. When the police arrived, Delia was hurling her massive frame against the metal front doors. One cop said it sounded like someone firing a cannon.

Delia slept through the night and was already up on Ward Three when I arrived the next morning. "Fuck your medication!" I heard her shout as I walked down the hall. "God is in me! God hears me! God says no medication!"

I got to Delia's door just as Miss Givens was coming out. "You ordered it," she said, jamming a juice dose and small cup of pills into my hands. "You get her to take it."

Medication consent laws are cumbersome but very necessary. After all, knowing what you're taking and why, what you can and cannot expect and all your other options, is just good, basic medicine and common sense. A rational person, it's assumed, should have control over what goes into his or her body.

With psychiatric patients, however, things aren't quite so clear-cut. The operative word here is "rational." Many mental patients need medication but they're either too deluded or thought-disordered to understand why. Now we're into the subject of giving medicine to people against their will.

As you might gather, this is a minefield area. There's no question about giving sedatives on an emergency basis if anyone is in personal danger. But that's only a one-time, situation-by-situation thing. Long-term treatment is another matter altogether.

Competence, the ability to make reasonable decisions, is not, most people are surprised to learn, a psychiatric decision but strictly a legal one. I cannot declare you incompetent. That's left to a judge. And, as I'd discovered with Juan Cruz, this can be a lengthy process.

So, while we waited for her court date, the staff was left to deal with Delia Davis. We knew we either had to keep her snowed twenty-four hours a day or get creative. Something had to be done. Delia was tearing the place apart.

As soon as each sedative dose wore off, she was up and charging around like an irate elephant. "God is king!" she'd shout and toss a chair across the room. Restraints were becoming a problem. Delia'd already shredded three sets of heavy leather ones. We were living under a true reign of terror. There wasn't a person, patient or staff, who didn't check both ways before venturing out into the hall.

If it hadn't been for Dr. Markham, we'd probably all have been dead inside a week.

V

"Tough case," Dr. Markham said at rounds. "Poor woman."

Just then, Delia Davis came thundering down the hall and began to bang on the conference room door. "Damnation to all sinners!" she shouted, over and over.

Until I heard security arrive, I was honestly frightened. Those hinges were really beginning to rattle. For an instant I contemplated whether I would shield Dr. Ashwin if the door gave way or merely dive headfirst under the table.

"We don't go to court for four days," I said as the Delia Davis/security guard battle moved slowly away. "I'm not sure what to do."

"And if she doesn't get some anticonvulsant medicine in her pretty soon," Glen Charles stated, "we're in for serious trouble."

"The family called this morning," Miss Givens added. "They want to know why we haven't done anything."

Everyone was silently staring at Dr. Markham with a "save us" look on our faces.

"Have you considered all your options?" he said after thinking a minute.

"We're beaten," I sighed dejectedly.

"She's a religious woman, right?" Dr. Markham asked.

"Pillar of the church," Glen Charles replied. "When she's on her lithium."

"Then we must enlist God's help," Dr. Markham said with a smile, his right index finger pointing heavenward.

TWENTY-ONE

OF GOD AND BASEBALL

I

"DELIA DAVIS, this is God speaking," the intercom announcement said. "I command you to take your medicine."

Miss Givens and I were watching Delia patrol the empty hall from a safe vantage in the nursing station. When God's voice came overhead, she stopped dead in her tracks. She looked in front of her. She looked behind her. Finally she looked up at the ceiling. When the same message was repeated, Delia's face burst into a glorious smile. "HALLELUJAH!" she shouted and headed toward us.

Instinctively, Miss Givens and I lurched backwards, each pulling a chair in front of us. But Delia Davis didn't come barging through the door. Instead she stood outside quietly.

With a mounting sense of hope I opened the top half of the Dutch door. "Yes, Delia," I said.

"I'm supposed to have my medication," she replied. "Orders from God."

Miss Givens had the stuff ready in a flash. "I guess you've been replaced," she said to me, handing Delia her pills.

235

"If there're any new orders," I added with a smile, "make sure He signs them."

While I wouldn't advocate supporting every patient's delusional system, with Delia Davis I think it was making the best of a bad situation. Plus, it worked like a charm. Twice each day for a week, Glen Charles made his way down to the paging operator's office and repeated his commands from on high. And twice each day Delia Davis dutifully obeyed.

We were a bit concerned about the effect God speaking on the PA system might have on the other patients. But we only heard one comment. It came from a resident on Ward Two. He'd asked a patient of his who was also troubled by messages from God if he'd heard the announcements. "Somebody's fooling you, Doc," the man was reported to have said. "That's Doctor Charles from Ward Three."

Inside of a week Delia Davis was under basic control. An occasional piece of furniture got tossed but it was nothing major. By two weeks she was back to normal.

The day Delia Davis was discharged, she passed Dr. Charles and me as we stood in the hallway.

"Goodbye, Doctor Seager," she said and shook my hand. Glen and I both wished her good luck. Just before leaving the ward, however, she turned one last time and looked at me. "You know," she said, "your friend sounds just like God."

II

There are, in my view, two basic forces in the universe, both of which are inviolate and not to be trifled with. The first are the laws of nature, gravity, $E=mc^2$, that kind of stuff. Second is baseball. I'm definitely suspect of anyone who tries to disparage or tarnish either. Men cannot travel faster than the speed of light. What goes up must come down. Baseballs were not meant to be hit under domed roofs by designated hitters who don't play in the field. I feel very strongly about these issues.

I mention baseball because as May became June, as the weather warmed and grass grew, that's where my thoughts turned as they had every year in spring.

Baseball season at our house meant two things: Little League and trading cards. In my life there have never been more satisfying times than those hours I'd spent watching my young sons standing on that diamond, mastering skills of the game I'd so loved as a child.

And baseball cards are the visual proof of all these memories. Each has a specific sentiment or feeling attached to it. Save a span of years in medical school and college, I've always been part of "The Hobby," as it's called. And I've taken my share of grief, especially from clerks at 7-Eleven counters. To the question, "Why would a grown man collect bubble gum cards?" my standard reply is this: How many things do you still own that you bought with your own money when you were eight?

Baseball cards taught me a lot of things about memories, about the importance of the past, but, interestingly, as my year on Ward Three drew to a close, they taught me even more about myself and about being a doctor.

It happened with one card in particular. Children, as I had, have a way of grabbing onto one baseball player and taking him as their own. For me that player was Al Springer, an outfielder from the fifties and early sixties, my "wonder years."

Al Springer wasn't a particularly good player and is remembered now basically for just one thing. He was the only man in baseball history to be hit by a pitched ball four times in one game. Maybe that's why I liked him. The fifth time he batted that afternoon, he jerked one over the wall. There's an allegory in there somewhere. At nine I thought so, anyway.

Being my favorite player, naturally I traded for all the Al Springer cards I could get. Which was fortunate. Especially after he became my patient.

During his years as a player, Al Springer had always been a little odd. Nothing serious mind you, mainly things only a true Spring-erphile would notice. During one televised game toward the end of his career, the camera panned to the outfield where, just prior to starting time, a lone player was dutifully signing autographs for a clutch of admiring young fans. A real slice of Americana everyone thought, except, perhaps, those boys who actually got the autographs. Mine read "Obey God."

A newspaper clipping I'd seen a few years back under the heading "Where are they now?" said Al Springer was down on his luck. Which was true. He'd been unlucky enough to come down with schizophrenia.

At first I didn't recognize him. Standing in the middle of our triage area floor he looked just like any other filth-ridden man, unshaven and grimy. As usual, two policemen were there, too. One guarding Al and the other filling out forms.

Then that dirt-covered man walked over to get a sip of water. It was a walk I'd seen a thousand times before. The slight hitch, the slow pace, he might just as well have been striding to the plate. I didn't even have to look at the hold papers.

"That's Al Springer," I said with an excitement unbefitting the occasion.

The two young cops looked up. "You know this guy?" one asked with mild surprise.

"Don't you?" I said, walking over to help Mr. Springer with the fountain. The policemen looked at me strangely.

"Al Springer played big-league ball," I said as he pushed my hand away and finished drinking on his own.

The cops seemed momentarily impressed, but it passed quickly. "He's been shagging flies on the moon lately," one of them said, and the other laughed.

I was suddenly angry but didn't reply. Instead, I took Al's hold papers and made arrangements to get him downstairs.

"Take two and hit to right, old-timer," the cops said as they left. Al didn't seem to notice. He was talking to the floor.

"That's Al Springer," I said to Miss Phipps, the PES nurse, as she left the nursing station to admit our new patient. "He played major-league ball."

Miss Phipps was back in ten seconds. She was fanning both hands in front of her face. "He's Mr. major-league shit pants now," she said, summoning help. "Get Mr. Springer into the shower," she said when another nurse arrived.

With a few minutes to spare I read Al's paperwork. He'd been arrested at a local softball park for peeing on the pitcher's mound during a women's championship game. No matter how far down you slide, I suppose, baseball never completely gets out of your system.

"Where do you want to admit your friend?" Miss Phipps asked. She had the phone cradled against her shoulder.

"Ward Three, of course," I replied.

"Ward Three's full," she said.

"I'll transfer someone," I said.

Miss Phipps looked at the clock. "At this time of night?"

"I'll push the bed myself," I said. And that's exactly what I did.

III

I had big plans for Al Springer. I saw this as a rare opportunity to repay some of the joy he'd given me. I was determined to make him well, regardless. What I should have said was regardless of whose feelings got hurt or how big an ass I made of myself.

I think I was buoyed by how much better Al looked in clean clothes, with all the twigs out of his hair. After two days on the ward you could have put a uniform on him and sent him out to center field.

I presented Al Springer's case at rounds that morning. "Doesn't he look terrific?" I said and, like the cops had in triage, everybody looked at me funny, including Dr. Markham, which was unusual.

"I mean compared to two days ago," I added. "The night he first came in. But, of course, you didn't see him then. He was a mess." I was rambling and knew it, so I shut up.

"Are you feeling okay?" Miss Givens asked.

I checked everyone's face again. "Sure," I bubbled. "I feel great. Why?"

"You're giddy," Miss Givens said. "Does this guy owe you money or something?"

"I'm the one who owes him," I said without thinking and the strange looks intensified.

"Does anyone understand what's happening here?" Miss Givens asked, shaking her head.

"A slight case of hero worship, I think," Glen Charles said.

"No, not at all," I protested. "It's just that I . . . I . . . ." I said, but couldn't finish. Glen was exactly right. "I just feel sorry for the guy," I said finally.

"We all do," Dr. Markham added. "Next case."

I couldn't tell if I was making any progress with Al Springer because for that entire first week he didn't say a single word to anyone. I knew he was getting his medications. I'd seen to that personally, making certain I was in the nursing station at the appropriate times and handing him the pills myself. After a while, this began to get on Miss Givens's nerves. "Don't you have anything better to do?" she finally said.

"Humor me," I said, passing Al his afternoon medicine.

"If you don't get out of my hair," Miss Givens snapped angrily, "I'll really humor you one."

I stopped giving Al Springer his pills, but I still kept coming to the nursing station at medication time just to keep an eye on things.

But the harder I tried, the more things I did for Al, the worse I felt. He just wasn't making any progress. Our interviews consisted of me exerting an exorbitant amount of energy just to get the guy to nod his head.

The staff started to get on my case a little, too. "You sleeping with this guy or what?" Dr. Lamb asked one day at rounds.

"I'm trying to do everything I can for the man," I said.

"Leave him be. He's a man on a mission," Glen Charles added, which made Dr. Ashwin laugh.

Again, Dr. Markham said nothing. In fact, I began to realize, he hadn't said much to me about Al Springer at all.

After three weeks of medication, recreation therapy, occupational therapy, and my personal service therapy, after all this and Al Springer was still mumbling to his shoes, I decided to deploy my ultimate weapon. It was something no baseball player could possibly resist.

The next morning my wife was curious when she saw me fumbling through my boxes of baseball cards an hour before leaving for work. "You going to trade with your little friends at the hospital?" she said sweetly.

"Very funny," I said, pulling out the prize and holding it to the light. "This is serious. This guy's my patient," I added, pointing to the 1959 Topps card.

"And you think seeing this old card will somehow jog Mr. Springer back to reality?" Linda asked.

"Guaranteed," I said, sliding the card into my shirt pocket. "I have this feeling."

"Call me before you make any trades with the older boys," Linda said at the door. "Remember, you paid good money for your cards."

Did I mention that my wife was also a comedienne?

I found Al Springer sitting in his room. I showed him the card, gently cradling it in my palms. "That's you, Mr. Springer," I said. "Remember?" Al Springer glanced at the card, then muttered something toward the floor.

I figured he just needed more time. Besides, rounds were about to begin. "Here," I said, propping the card on Al's nightstand. "You keep it. I have plenty."

Rounds began at ninish. I started with an update on Mr. Springer.

"Shouldn't this guy be at the state hospital?" Dr. Lamb said, stroking his recently acquired pitiful excuse for a beard. "He obviously needs locked placement."

Glen Charles sensed my rising anger and spoke before I blew up. "I think he's right, Steve," he said gently.

"Me, too," Dr. Ashwin agreed.

I turned to Dr. Markham. "Do you agree?" I asked pathetically.

"What do you think is best for Mr. Springer?" Dr. Markham said.

Great, I thought, the heat was off. "Give me another week," I said brightly. None of them knew about the baseball card. In seven days, I was certain, I'd be having the last laugh.

"Another week is fine," Dr. Markham said. "But why not get started on conservatorship papers anyway," he added. "Just in case."

"No problem," I said confidently.

I checked Al Springer's room before I left for home that night. The card was still where I'd left it.

IV

If I ever doubted the power of this boyhood baseball-card-trading mystique, when Al Springer spoke the next morning, it was forever erased.

He was waiting for me at the door of his room when I walked onto the ward. Immediately I sensed something different about him.

Looking me straight in the eye, he held out a closed hand. "Keep this fucking shit out of here," he said distinctly as tiny bits of shredded cardboard trickled from his palm to the floor.

"The state hospital will be fine," I said when Al Springer's name came up at Friday's rounds.

"What happened?" Dr. Ashwin asked.

"I came to my senses," I said hurriedly, anxious to move on.

Then everyone was silent for a while. "Can you get in touch with your anger?" Dr. Markham said to me quietly.

Inside I was raging like a fireball. "I'm not angry," I lied weakly.

"You'd better let go of your chair arms, anyway," Dr. Lamb said. "Before you shoot them through the ceiling."

He was right. I had my chair in a real death grip. I looked down, then sort of slumped.

"Let me give you some advice, Steve," Dr. Markham said. "Take it for what it's worth. You're angry because you did everything in your power for this man and he didn't get better. Not only that," he added, "he wasn't even grateful for the effort."

Dr. Markham leaned forward a little. "I know you experienced this with your ER patients," he said, "but not as keenly. The hurt wasn't as deep. That's the great thing about psychiatry. You have the wonderful opportunity to get involved. To truly feel elation and dejection. It's a specialty that deals with life. Live your feelings. Work through them. Experience them. Then afford that same gift to your patients. Don't expect gratitude," he added, staring me straight in the eye. "Just being part of this beautiful mess is thanks enough."

"Sorry about your baseball card," Dr. Ashwin said, breaking the long silence after Dr. Markham stopped speaking.

"You knew?" I said.

Anita nodded her head, as did everyone around the table.

"Hey," Glen Charles said. "I heard this Springer guy was pretty much of an asshole back in his playing days, too."

I'm not sure what happened during rounds that morning, but now, on a little reflection, I think I began to become a psychiatrist.

V

And then it was over. I'd been so wrapped up with Al Springer and baseball and Ward Three that the time just went by. I'd probably still be there if Miss Givens hadn't said something. "Where you going to be next Monday?" she said after Friday rounds.

I wasn't sure where she was going. "Right here, of course," I said. "Why?"

She looked at Glen Charles and Anita Ashwin who were also in the nursing station. Then she bonked the side of her head with her hand. "You take too many fast balls in the bean or something?" she said with a laugh.

I was a little slow on the uptake that day. "What's she talking about?" I asked Glen, who simply pointed at a calendar hanging on the wall. His finger was aimed at July first.

"Holy shit," was all I could say. The year was over. Next Monday I would move downstairs to the adult outpatient department for six months and actually be expected to do therapy. Suddenly I was scared to death.

"I'm not ready," I said, looking up and down the familiar halls of Ward Three. "I need more time. I don't know anything."

"You'll do fine," Anita said. "I'll be around. If you run into trouble, call me." I found great comfort in that, but the flip side of Dr. Ashwin's statement gave me a chill. If Anita's and my years were ending and we were staying, that meant Glen Charles was leaving for good.

"Hey, we'll see each other," Glen said. "We're friends, remember?" And it's true—we were.

I looked around to say something to Miss Givens, but she'd disappeared. Dr. Markham wasn't in sight, either. I looked at the calendar again just to be sure. "Huh," I sighed.

I could lie and say we all had an emotion-packed, meaningful farewell that last day on Ward Three. I could lie, too, and say I spent my final day contemplating everything I'd learned and reminiscing about the people I'd met. But that wouldn't be true, either. I was much too nervous thinking about what I would say to all my new patients on Monday. As goodbyes went, that short conversation in the nursing station had pretty much been it.

I finished up my paperwork around five that night. Dr. Markham and Miss Givens had gone home. Dr. Ashwin and Glen Charles were somewhere else in the building. I could hear the evening nurses chatting quietly in the dayroom.

I'd packed a few personal things into a small box as I scanned my office one last time before closing and locking the door. Mine were the only steps in the hallway.

I stood in front of the empty nursing station and briefly stared in through the glass. My eye was drawn to Singer Carlysle's picture on the bulletin board. "You'll sure have some story to tell about the day you were born," I whispered quietly and gave the photo a small goodbye wave.

Turning to leave, I passed by the conference room door. The tile outside was completely clean now, that last fleck of Dr. Singh's blood having long since eroded away. I stopped to linger for a moment.

"He was a fine man, sir," Ben Smith said, coming up behind me. His mops were locked in the closet, his day at an end. I had been too engrossed in thought to hear his approach.

"Yes, Ben, he was," I sighed, looking up from the floor. "I know I'll never forget him."

"None of us will, sir," Ben said, reaching out to shake my hand. "And none of us up here will forget you, either." That afternoon I'd promised myself I wasn't going to break down when I left Ward Three, but now I was none too sure about keeping that vow.

"Thanks, Ben," I said, fighting back a tear. Finally, I couldn't control the emotion welling inside me. I set down my box of office things and pulled Ben into an embrace. And Ben hugged me back.

"Take care of yourself, boy," he said quietly, then, with a nervous laugh, broke free and stood back. He was straightening his shirt. "Wouldn't do for anyone to see two grown men behaving like this," he said with a firm nod.

I said I agreed and picked up my box. "Don't be no stranger now, sir," Ben said as I turned and headed for the main door.

"Don't worry," I called back. "I know where you live."

There was a young man standing at the door leading into the main corridor. He was gazing through the little window. He stepped aside as I approached and for a moment we stood face to face. He had that Al Springer-Martin Braga-2.5 million schizophrenics' look in his eyes.

I reached inside my box and pulled out a red flower I'd picked at lunch and intended to give to my wife.

"I'm sorry," I said, handing it to the man.

Then I opened the door, walked outside, rode downstairs, and went home.

VI

I dropped by the ward that July first morning. I'd decided I couldn't leave without saying goodbye to Miss Givens. As I walked into the nursing station I saw a pixie-cute young woman with blonde hair wearing a starched white lab coat, standing nervously in the corner. Miss Givens was beside me.

"She your new intern?" I asked.

"Afraid so," Miss Givens replied.

"Won't last a week," we both said, then laughed.

AFTERWORD

As I SAID, I am now nearing the end of my formal psychiatric training. I'm at the stage Glen Charles was when I first met him.

Glen finished his time at County General that final day in June and, as expected, took an offer to join a large Beverly Hills private practice. True to his word, he did stay in touch. The last time we had lunch, however, he mentioned a growing dissatisfaction with his job and even hinted that he might like to return to County General as an attending.

Anita Ashwin completed her residency last year and moved to New York City for two years of child-psychiatry specialty work. I received a letter from her recently. She and her husband are thinking about having a baby.

Dr. Markham and Miss Givens are still up on Ward Three, and as each new group of interns and residents first rotates through there, I see them at lunch with those same confused looks on their faces.

The Bin is still The Bin and the county board is still the county board. A month ago, they proposed another round of sweeping cuts in our mental health budget. As of now, no formal response is in the offing.

As for me, I'm not sure what I'll do when I'm done at The Bin. But I do know this: When it comes time to decide, I'll have lots of good advice. My lawn chair still gets regular use at Minnie Osbourne's gravesite.

Ben Smith died quietly in his sleep last April.